Lecture Notes in Computer Science　　11148

Commenced Publication in 1973
Founding and Former Series Editors:
Gerhard Goos, Juris Hartmanis, and Jan van Leeuwen

More information about this series at http://www.springer.com/series/7409

Siuly Siuly · Ickjai Lee
Zhisheng Huang · Rui Zhou
Hua Wang · Wei Xiang (Eds.)

Health Information Science

7th International Conference, HIS 2018
Cairns, QLD, Australia, October 5–7, 2018
Proceedings

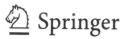

Springer

Editors
Siuly Siuly
Victoria University
Footscray, VIC
Australia

Ickjai Lee ⓘ
James Cook University
Cairns, QLD
Australia

Zhisheng Huang
Vrije University of Amsterdam
Amsterdam
The Netherlands

Rui Zhou ⓘ
Swinburne University of Technology
Hawthorn, VIC
Australia

Hua Wang ⓘ
Victoria University
Footscray, VIC
Australia

Wei Xiang
James Cook University
Cairns, QLD
Australia

ISSN 0302-9743   ISSN 1611-3349   (electronic)
Lecture Notes in Computer Science
ISBN 978-3-030-01077-5   ISBN 978-3-030-01078-2   (eBook)
https://doi.org/10.1007/978-3-030-01078-2

Library of Congress Control Number: 2018955284

LNCS Sublibrary: SL3 – Information Systems and Applications, incl. Internet/Web, and HCI

This Springer imprint is published by the registered company Springer Nature Switzerland AG
The registered company address is: Gewerbestrasse 11, 6330 Cham, Switzerland

Preface

The International Conference Series on Health Information Science (HIS) provides a forum for disseminating and exchanging multidisciplinary research results in computer science/information technology and health science and services. It covers all aspects of health information sciences and systems that support health information management and health service delivery.

The 7th International Conference on Health Information Science (HIS 2018) was held in Cairns, Queensland, Australia, during October 5–7, 2018. Founded in April 2012 as the International Conference on Health Information Science and Their Applications, the conference continues to grow to include an ever-broader scope of activities. The main goal of these events is to provide international scientific forums for researchers to exchange new ideas in a number of fields that interact in depth through discussions with their peers from around the world. The scope of the conference includes: (1) medical/health/biomedicine information resources, such as patient medical records, devices and equipments, software and tools to capture, store, retrieve, process, analyze, and optimize the use of information in the health domain; (2) data management, data mining, and knowledge discovery, all of which play a key role in decision-making, management of public health, examination of standards, privacy and security issues; (3) computer visualization and artificial intelligence for computer-aided diagnosis; and (4) development of new architectures and applications for health information systems.

The conference solicited and gathered technical research submissions related to all aspects of the conference scope. All the submitted papers in the proceeding were peer reviewed by at least three international experts drawn from the Program Committee. After the rigorous peer-review process, a total of 13 full papers and five short papers among 43 submissions were selected on the basis of originality, significance, and clarity and were accepted for publication in the proceedings. The authors were from Australia, Bangladesh, China, Finland, Russia, and The Netherlands. Some authors were invited to submit extended versions of their papers to a special issue of the *Health Information Science and System* journal published by Springer.

The high quality of the program – guaranteed by the presence of an unparalleled number of internationally recognized top experts – in reflected the contents of the proceeding. The conference was therefore a unique event, where attendees were able to appreciate the latest results in their field of expertise, and to acquire additional knowledge in other fields. The program was structured to favor interactions among attendees coming from many different areas, scientifically and geographically, from academia and from industry.

We would like to sincerely thank our keynote and invited speaker:

– Professor Fernando Martin-Sanchez, FACMI, FACHI, CHIA, FIAHSI, Instituto de Salud Carlos III, Spain

Our thanks also go to the host organization, James Cook University, Australia. Finally, we acknowledge all those who contributed to the success of HIS 2018 but whose names are not listed here.

October 2018

Siuly Siuly
Ickjai Lee
Zhisheng Huang
Rui Zhou
Hua Wang
Wei Xiang

Organization

General Co-chairs

Yanchun Zhang   Victoria University, Australia and Fudan University, China
Wei Xiang   James Cook University, Australia
Uwe Aickelin   University of Melbourne, Australia

Program Co-chairs

Siuly Siuly   Victoria University, Australia
Ickjai Lee   James Cook University, Australia
Zhisheng Huang   Vrije Universiteit Amsterdam, The Netherlands

Conference Organization Chair

Hua Wang   Victoria University, Australia

Publicity Co-chairs

Juanying Xie   Shaanxi Normal University, China
Ji Zhang   University of Southern Queensland, Australia

Publication Chair

Rui Zhou   Swinburne University of Technology, Australia

Local Arrangements Chair

Lei Lei   James Cook University, Australia
Jiangang Ma   James Cook University, Australia

Webmaster

Sarathkumar Rangarajan   Victoria University, Australia

Program Committee

Uwe Aickelin   University of Melbourne, Australia
Omer Faruk Alçin   Bingöl University, Turkey
Jiang Bian   University of Florida, USA
Fei Chen   South University of Science and Technology, China

Soon Ae Chun	The City University of New York, USA
James Cimino	National Institutes of Health, USA
Licong Cui	University of Kentucky, USA
Grazziela Figueredo	University of Nottingham, UK
Yanhui Guo	University of Illinois Springfield, USA
Zhisheng Huang	Vrije Universiteit Amsterdam, The Netherlands
Du Huynh	University of Western Australia, Australia
Xia Jing	Ohio University, USA
Enamul Kabir	University of Southern Queensland, Australia
Ickjai Lee	James Cook University, Australia
Gang Luo	University of Washington, USA
Zhiyuan Luo	Royal Holloway, University of London, UK
Fernando Martin-Sanchez	Instituto de Salud Carlos III, Spain
Bridget Mcinnes	Virginia Commonwealth University, USA
Fleur Mougin	ERIAS, INSERM, U1219, Université de Bordeaux, France
Trina Myers	James Cook University, Australia
William Song	Dalarna University, Sweden
Weiqing Sun	University of Toledo, USA
Xiaohui Tao	University of Southern Queensland, Australia
Pasupathy Vimalachandran	Victoria University, Australia
Hua Wang	Victoria University, Australia
Jimin Wen	Guilin University of Electronic Technology, China
Wei Xiang	James Cook University, Australia
Ji Zhang	University of Southern Queensland, Australia
Rui Zhou	Swinburne University of Technology, Australia
Fengfeng Zhou	Jilin University, China

Additional Reviewers

Huang, Yan
Li, Xiaojin
Tao, Shiqiang
Wu, Xi
Yang, Xi
Zeng, Ningzhou
Zhu, Wei

Contents

Data Management, Data Mining, and Knowledge Discovery Mining

Development of New Architectures and Applications

Medical, Health, Biomedicine Information

Perceptions and Experiences of General Practice Users About MyHealthRecord

Urooj Raza Khan[1(✉)], Tanveer A. Zia[1], Chris Pearce[2],
and Kaushalya Perera[1]

[1] School of Computing and Mathematics,
Charles Sturt University, Wagga Wagga, NSW 2678, Australia
urazakhan@csu.edu.au
[2] The University of Melbourne, Melbourne, Australia

Abstract. Background: It is widely expected in Australia that digital health solutions such as MyHealthRecord (MyHR) have vast potential to enable easier, safer and faster patientcare. Being the gateway to the health system, the general practice environment has been one of the target areas for MyHR adoption. Aim: This doctoral qualitative research aims to investigate MyHR adoption in the general practices of Victoria and explore its users' views/experiences. Method: This paper presents the survey results, a component of the study which was distributed in 2017 to general practices and its consumers. The survey was designed based on research questions to gain users views, experiences and ideas for improving adoption. Findings: There were 230 valid responses which included 179 consumers/patients and 51 healthcare providers/staff members. Results shows users appreciate that using MyHR contributes to easier and faster patientcare but correlation with the improved safety aspect is not clearly understood. Most of respondents rated their MyHR experience as never heard/good/excellent/neutral, however, there were also few ratings of poor/very poor experience. Majority were interested in encouraging the usage of MyHR and shared their ideas for improvements. Conclusion: There is a strong need to create more awareness and education about the MyHR system and its benefits.

Keywords: Digital health · MyHealthRecord · MyHR · PCEHR
General practice

1 Introduction

Driven by the need of changing population demographics, financial implications, workforce shortages, health service provision, advancement in medical technologies and their impact on healthcare delivery, digital health (DH) is the focus of many countries, including Australia [1]. The MyHealthRecord (MyHR), formerly known as the Personally Controlled Electronic Health Record (launched in 2012) was envisaged as the foundation of Australia's digital health infrastructure [2] with the belief that centralising fragmented medical records using MyHR will simplify the patient journey. It is designed to deliver better healthcare, enable informed consumer decision making and reduce healthcare costs [3, 4]. The MyHR national approach received support from

© Springer Nature Switzerland AG 2018
S. Siuly et al. (Eds.): HIS 2018, LNCS 11148, pp. 3–16, 2018.
https://doi.org/10.1007/978-3-030-01078-2_1

the Australian public, health experts [3, 5] and government [6]. Australia had the necessary infrastructure and had the required technological foundation with 95% of GPs using clinical information systems (CIS) and most public hospitals in various stages of digitization [3]. However, despite of all the support, driving factors and readiness, implementation of any DH solution remains a complex process [7]. MyHR implementation generally faced criticisms for slow uptake due to its opt-in model, usability issues, privacy concerns and security risks by stakeholders, local healthcare IT experts and researchers [3].

Most Australians see their General Practitioner (GP), thus they act as gateway to the health system [8, 9] and have an essential role in providing information to MyHR. A GP readiness report indicated in 2011 that GPs were generally positive about this system if it was to facilitate their ability to share and communicate their patient information. The challenge noted for adoption was the need of additional time required by GPs to participate [10]. According to latest MyHR statistics, 6,311 general practices signed up for the MyHR aided by the government eHealth Practice Incentives Programme (ePIP), but there are only 1,499,129 health summaries uploaded so far [11], indicating low usage. In an attempt to improve adoption, a policy intervention was also made in 2016, linking usage of system with eHealth incentives for practices [12]. This has initiated a change in the culturally complex general practice environment [13]. The degree and impact of this change is little known [14, 15]. A doctoral research project commenced an investigation in this space with an aim to explore MyHR adoption in general practices, identify its impacts and understand its users acceptance factors. Scope of study was limited to the state of Victoria only due to time and resources constraints. Literature review was conducted systematically, and data were collected in the field with the help of interviews, surveys and observations. This paper presents findings of the survey that gathered users' perspectives and experiences in using MyHR.

2 Background

To define MyHR, it is a hybrid health information system integrating web based Personal Health Records (PHR) with clinical electronic health record systems, enabling consumers and healthcare providers to access health information through a platform with shared responsibilities and mixed governance model [16]. It is a centralized serviced accessible to consumers and healthcare providers. Consumers can register to it either themselves through the consumers portal or through their healthcare providers. Healthcare providers have access to MyHR through their clinical information system (CIS), where they can register patients and upload their health summaries. This MyHR-CIS integration implementation occurs when healthcare providers/general practices register themselves for eHealth incentives. At present, the system is opt-out: patients/consumers are registered to the system only when interested. GPs usually are presented with CIS patient record, which they review with the patient for any required updates and then upload shared health summaries (SHS) to MyHR. Consumers are also able add some information about their health condition/s and/or update access control of their records [4, 17–19].

A literature review going back five years [15] shows that MyHR evaluation has been the focus of some research community members and industry experts. Limited knowledge and community unawareness of the system and its low benefits delivery/impacts were generally noted [19–25]. Need of increased trust on system, clarifications on regulations, standards, and addressing of privacy and security concerns was identified [17, 24, 26]. System usability issues were reported in consumer portal [27–29] along with complex CIS-MyHR implementations [20, 24], despite of given effective support [30]. Healthcare providers/clinicians had their own reservations with change in workflow [4, 30–32], data quality [33] and personal control given to patients in the system [34], resulting lack of interest among clinicians [21]. MyHR review was called in by the government to examine the associated issues resulting in PCEHR rebranding and opt-out approach trials [5].

3   Method

As part of qualitative case study research, a survey was developed for both staff and patients. We aimed to gain their input about their experiences and views about MyHR and its potential impacts including how to encourage adoption. Ethical approval for this study was granted by the Faculty of Business, Justice and Behavioural Sciences Human Research Ethics Committee of Charles Sturt University. Survey distribution (Mar-Nov 2017) was done using an online and hard copy form. The hard copy form was distributed in two medical centers and online form was shared via social media, consumer health forum (HIC) and AMA (Victoria) newsletter. This resulted in reaching an audience of approximately 1200 people, attracting 271 responses.

Details of the survey questions and given options are described below in results section along with the responses of healthcare professionals and patients:

4   Results

Out of 271 responses received, 230 were found valid and complete; 179 were surveys by patients/consumers and 51 by healthcare professionals (Fig. 1).

4.1   Demographics

The survey gathered basic demographic details at the start such as: age, gender, computer skills and how they heard about the research. They were given option to define their connection to general practice, either as patients or healthcare professional. Based on their selection, further questions were shown, e.g. patients were asked about how often they visit a GP, their accessibility to internet, if/how they are registered with MyHR, etc. Healthcare professionals were given option to further identify their role in general practice, e.g. GP, nurse, admin/reception, practice manager etc. and if they uploaded any health summaries or interacted with MyHR in some way.

Patients/Consumers: 179 respondents, broken up into age ranges: 18–24 (8), 25–34 (53), 35–54 (73) and 55 or over (45). Females (131) and males (48) with mostly

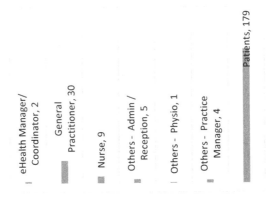

Fig. 1. Survey responses by roles

reporting excellent computer skills[1] (97) and others as moderate[2] (63) to good[3] (19) skills. The majority visited their GP either a couple of times a year or once a month. Most of their health records were maintained at the GP (147), some maintained their records themselves (56) and there were 4 patients/consumers who had eHealth records. 164 had access to internet all the time and others had access once or twice a week, within a day, or within an hour.

Healthcare Providers. The survey received 51 responses from various roles among general practice staff. It included 30 general practitioners, 9 nurses, 4 practice managers, 5 admin/reception, 2 eHealth coordinators and 1 physiotherapist. The majority of were aged 35–54, with 29 females and 22 males. Most reported to have excellent, moderate and good computer skills to navigate websites, perform online transactions and use Office software. These respondents were all across the State from 25 different postcodes around Melbourne suburbs and regional Victoria. Most of these practices were 6–10 years old medical centers with GPs and allied health professionals; where respondents had been working there for 1–5 years. On average, these practices attended 100–250 patients per day, where GP respondents sees 15–20 patients per session.

4.2   Interaction with MyHR

Before asking respondents' views/experiences, we enquired about their level of interaction with MyHR. To identify interactions, patients were asked if they were registered with MyHR and how they learned about it. Healthcare professionals were asked if their practice was registered with MyHR and specify the number of health summaries uploaded. Overall response indicated only 91/230 participants had interacted with MyHR in some way (Table 1).

---

[1] Excellent (e.g. can perform online transactions and use Office and other softwares).

[2] Moderate (e.g. can navigate into websites).

[3] Good (e.g. can navigate into websites and perform online transactions).

Table 1. Survey respondents' interaction with MyHR

Survey respondents	Interacted: Yes	Interacted: No	Total
Patients	52	127	179
GPs	26	4	30
Nurses	4	5	9
Practice Managers	4	0	4
eHealth roles	2	0	2
Admin/Reception	3	2	5
Physiotherapist	0	1	1
TOTAL	91	139	230

Patients/Consumers. 52 respondents were registered with MyHR either by their healthcare provider (hospital (3) and medical practice (20)) or themselves (29). The majority reported that they entered their health record details themselves along with their healthcare providers. A variety of sources were noted when they were asked about how they learnt about MyHR including: GP/hospital, via this or prior similar research, or involved through their work.

Healthcare Providers. Out of 51 respondents, 39 worked in a practice registered with MyHR. 11 respondents were not aware of how many summaries had been uploaded by their practice whereas others reported upload of 10 to 400 health summaries so far to MyHR.

4.3   Perspectives About MyHR Potential Impacts

The survey attempted to gather respondents' views about MyHR exploring if it was able to facilitate easier, faster and safer patient care. Rating scale options including more (M), about the same (S), less (L) and don't know (D) were used. Overall respondents believed the MyHR could potentially enable easier and faster patient care but they were not sure about it providing safer patient care (Table 2).

   Patients/Consumers rated 'more/much more' among the two categories of MyHR being able to offer faster and easier patient care, even though majority of the patient respondents (127) were not registered with MyHR.

   Healthcare Providers ratings breakdown shows:

- GPs thinks patient care may be faster but effect on being easier and safer would remain about the same.
- Nurses selection indicated patient care would become easier, faster and safer.
- Practice managers believed patient care might become easier and offer safety but not faster.
- eHealth roles thought MyHR might result more or less impact on easier and faster patient care but safety would be more or about the same.
- Admin respondents selected more for easier, faster and safer patient care with MyHR.

Table 2. Perspective on MyHR potential impacts on the patient care

Survey respondents	Patients	GPs	Nurses	Practice Managers	eHealth roles	Admin/Reception	Physio therapist	Total
Easier								
M	80	8	5	3	1	3	0	100
S	25	11	1	1	0	1	0	39
L	5	6	0	0	1	1	0	13
D	69	5	3	0	0	0	1	78
Total	179	30	9	4	2	5	1	230
Faster								
M	78	12	5	1	1	4	0	101
S	27	7	2	3	0	1	0	40
L	4	6	0	0	1	0	0	11
D	70	5	2	0	0	0	1	78
Total	179	30	9	4	2	5	1	230
Safer								
M	55	7	4	2	1	3	0	72
S	36	12	3	2	1	0	0	54
L	14	6	0	0	0	2	0	22
D	74	5	2	0	0	0	1	82
Total	179	30	9	4	2	5	1	230

- Physiotherapist respondents had no idea about these categories of potential patient care impacts.

4.4 Experience Using MyHR

The survey asked the respondents to rate their overall experience of using MyHR, with options of: excellent, good, neutral, poor, very poor, never used. The majority had not heard/used MyHR (150), with second highest ranking of excellent/good (33) or neutral experience (30) (Table 3).

Patients/Consumers. 134 out of 179 claimed to have not used it personally; 7 out of these 134 were registered but not used indicating that they might have been registered either by their healthcare provider or family/someone else. The rest of the 45 respondents registered with MyHR rated their experience as excellent/good (5/18), neutral (14) or poor/very poor (3/5).

Healthcare Providers experience in using MyHR gave mixed results, with neutral (16), good/excellent (10) and poor/very poor (9). Analysing the breakdown by roles shows that

- 7 out of 30 GPs and 5 out of 9 nurses' respondents never used it themselves. Most of other GPs (11) and nurses (3) rated their experience with MyHR neutral. There were 7 GPs and 1 nurses marking their experience as excellent/good whereas 5 GPs rated it as poor/very poor.

Table 3. Experience with MyHR

Survey respondents	Excellent/good	Neutral	Poor/very poor	Never heard/used	Total
Patients	23	14	8	134	179
GPs	7	11	5	7	30
Nurses	1	3	0	5	9
Practice Managers	2	1	1	0	4
eHealth roles	0	0	2	0	2
Admin/Reception	0	1	0	4	5
Physiotherapist	0	0	1	0	1
TOTAL	33	30	17	150	230

- Out of 4 practice managers 2 rated it as good, 1 neutral and 1 poor. Majority of the admin/reception (4) had not used it personally and 1 rated it as neutral.
- 2 eHealth roles and 1 physiotherapist rated their experience as poor/very poor.

Respondents were next asked to describe their experience. Patients were given an open text input box to comment. Patients who never experienced/used MyHR were also asked the reason. Healthcare professionals were given four input boxes in the categories of: strengths, weakness, opportunities and threats. All these responses were gathered, subjected to thematic analysis and grouped as four main themes (Fig. 2):

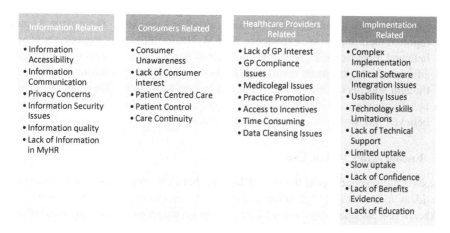

Fig. 2. MyHR views and experiences of survey respondents

(a) **Information related**. Four main streams about accessibility, security, communication and quality of health information were highlighted. Both healthcare professionals and patients strongly expressed their need for health information accessibility that they expected to achieve with MyHR. Being able to communicate information to other care givers about the patients using MyHR was also part of the expectation of some health care providers. At the same time, concerns were raised about information quality and content unavailability in MyHR records by both types of respondents. Information privacy and security issues were also elevated by survey participants.

(b) **Consumer related**. Lack of consumer awareness and interest was highly noted in the survey responses. Healthcare professionals emphasized on attaining potentially patient centered and care continuity with the use of MyHR. One healthcare professional praised the patient control that MyHR brings enabling patients of better health management. Others pointed out concerns about this patient control feature as it would result in patients withholding information, resulting in lack of confidence in MyHR record.

(c) **Healthcare Providers related**. General practices were found to be inclined towards MyHR implementation for being up-to-date with modern technology and to gain eHealth incentives. Some also seemed to be using it for their practice promotion and marketing, creating awareness in a way among their patients and staff. Some patient surveys indicated they were keen for MyHR but experienced lack of interest by their GPs. Healthcare providers also noted this issue of GP compliance to MyHR tasks. The perception of MyHR being time consuming was mentioned often by healthcare professionals. It was realized that data cleansing for MyHR uploads was an ongoing issue but also noted as an opportunity to clean up their records. Medicolegal issues were also mentioned number of times in the surveys causing confusion among GPs.

(d) **Implementation related**. Many healthcare professionals labelled MyHR implementation as complex and limited. They experienced issues in CIS integration, technical support, usability and connecting other caregivers. Some patients also reported their unpleasant experience with MyHR usability in consumer portal and believed their technological skills limitations had not being considered. Lack of education was the most mentioned factor by healthcare professionals that they thought was resulting in slow uptake and lack of confidence. There was no actual benefit delivery evidence on surface yet and some healthcare professionals believed this was contributing in slow uptake too.

4.5   Encouraging MyHR Use

We asked the respondents if the use of MyHR should be encouraged and what were their ideas to encourage it. Overall responses showed both consumers/patients and healthcare professionals (130 out of 230 surveys) were interested in encouraging the use of MyHR whereas 87 were not sure and 13 did not think MyHR should be promoted (Fig. 3).

Survey 130 respondents shared their ideas about how MyHR use should be encouraged and are summarized into four themes below (Fig. 4):

(a) **Education and Training** (Fig. 5) for general practitioners and other staff working in this space was the most highly mentioned suggestion. They were seeking more knowledge and information about how MyHR works and how best it can be used with convenience. With more MyHR knowledge, it would help them to clarify their concerns and make them comfortable to communicate it to their patients. An

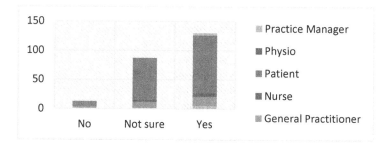

Fig. 3. Should MyHR use be encouraged?

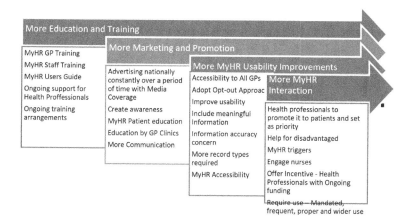

Fig. 4. Summary of ideas to encourage MyHR in General practices

ongoing arrangement for the training and its funding was believed to be vital. The training should also provide a detailed user guide for different professions involved at different levels of knowledge.

(b) **Marketing and Promotion** (Fig. 6) need was clearly identified to inform patients and create awareness in the community about significance of MyHR. Survey respondents highlighted variety of ideas along the lines of MyHR patient education, more communication and advertising. The majority believed education to patients by their GPs would be more effective. Information obtained via other staff in the GP clinic would also help. Advertising nationally and constantly over a period of time using social and other forms of media would be beneficial. More communication to patients was suggested using different sources, webinars, social media, posters, flyers, information sessions, in different languages and mail by their GP clinics. Showcasing real MyHR users and how it helped them must be identified and shared publicly to highlight its significance.

(c) **MyHR usability improvements** (Fig. 7) were suggested by survey respondents to encourage the use. It includes making MyHR more accessible through different platforms and to all GPs, as there were patients who wanted to use MyHR but

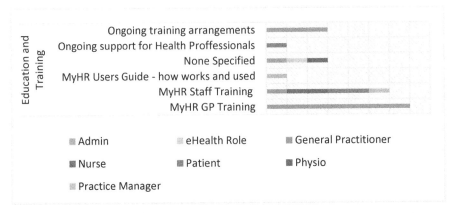

Fig. 5. Theme 1, More Education - Ideas to encourage MyHR in General practices

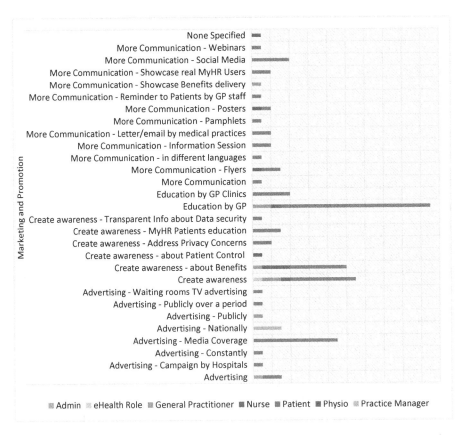

Fig. 6. Theme 2, More Marketing promotion - Ideas to encourage MyHR in General practices

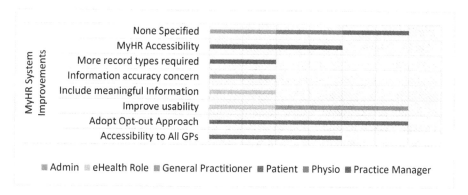

Fig. 7. Theme 3, More system improvements - Ideas to encourage MyHR in General practices

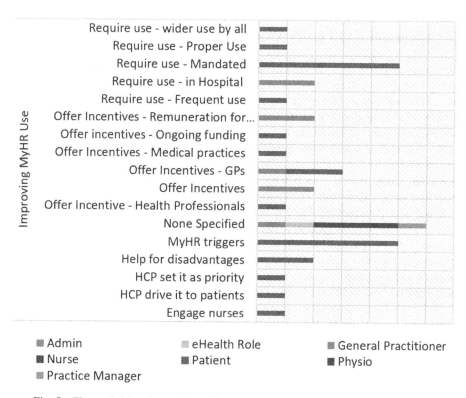

Fig. 8. Theme 4, More interaction - Ideas to encourage MyHR in General practices

could not. Many patients supported opt-out approach for MyHR. Need of enhancing usability was also highlighted along with inclusion of more record types and meaningful. Many patients supported opt-out approach for MyHR. Need of enhancing usability was also highlighted along with inclusion of more record types and meaningful information. There were also information accuracy concerns raised due to MyHR patient control and the consequences of information withholding.

(d) **MyHR interaction** (Fig. 8) and use was required more frequently, widely and constantly according to survey responses. Many patients' respondents suggested to make this system use mandated for health professionals, set it as their priority and drive it to patients. Others believed offering incentives and ongoing funding to health professionals would encourage the use. There was also a suggestion to engage nurses in improving MyHR use at the clinics. Patients highlighted that there were community members who could benefit from this system but require assistance in using and accessing technology, considering their needs was also vital. Some health conditions including chronic illness, seniors and younger communities were believed to be more of a trigger for MyHR use frequently and advantageously.

5 Conclusion and Future Work

The survey response of 23% was encouraging for a survey of this nature – distributed widely with no incentives. It provides information beneficial to understand the current views and experiences of MyHR users in general practice environment. Among these participants, the majority were females (70%) and were aged 35–54 with good to moderate computer skills. Many had interacted with MyHR in different ways. Views among consumers/patient participants captured a picture that demonstrates their perception of MyHR being able to facilitate easy and fast patient care. Healthcare providers had mixed views about potential impacts of MyHR as a way to enable easier, faster and safer patient care. The majority (65%) did not experience MyHR, but there were some respondents reporting excellent/good (14%) or neutral (13%) using this system. The views and experiences shared by participants were mainly around system unawareness, low level of interaction and unaddressed concerns of clinicians related to renumeration, quality and privacy of information. 57% proposed encouraging MyHR adoption and suggested to have more user education, more marketing, more usability improvements and more system use for better outcomes.

Although these survey findings are of MyHR adoption in Victoria, the results reflect vital insights for MyHR adoption in general. Statistics shows Victoria is one of the four major contributor of health summaries (SHS) in the system at present, with 20% of total patients' registrations and 23% of total general practices participation [35]. Hence in light of above findings, this paper suggests the system operator should offer more education and awareness opportunities for its users at different levels. Their perception needs to be aligned with the aimed objectives of the system; that it can offer safe, easier and faster patient care. There is also a need to increase interaction with the system to minimize fear of unknown and improve quality of records.

In future work, the survey results will be merged with a case study report to show insights of MyHR integration in general practice environment and recommendations to improve adoption.

References

1. Wickramasinghe, N., Schaffer, J.: Realizing value driven e-health solutions. Report for IBM, Washington (2010)
2. Department of Health and Ageing: PCEHR Annual Report 2012–2013 (2013). http://www.health.gov.au/internet/main/publishing.nsf/Content/PCEHR-system-operator-annual-report2012-2013
3. Xu, J., Gao, X., Sorwar, G., Croll, P.: Implementation of E-health record systems in Australia. Int. Technol. Manag. Rev. 3(2), 92–104 (2013)
4. Pearce, C., Bainbridge, M.: A personally controlled electronic health record for Australia. J. Am. Med. Inform. Assoc. 21(4), 707–713 (2014)
5. Fry, C.L., Spriggs, M., Arnold, M., Pearce, C.: Unresolved ethical challenges for the australian personally controlled electronic health record (PCEHR) system: key informant interview findings. AJOB Empir. Bioeth. Prespectives Eval. 5(4), 30–36 (2014)
6. Australia Digital Health Agency: Australia's national digital health strategy 2018–2022 (2017)
7. Gajanayake, R., Sahama, T., Iannella, R.: The role of perceived usefulness and attitude on electronic health record acceptance. In: IEEE 15th International Conference on e-Health Networking, Applications & Services (Healthcom), 2013, pp. 388–393 (2014)
8. Australian Bureau of Statistics: Patient experiences in Australia: summary of findings, 2014–15 (2015). http://www.abs.gov.au/AUSSTATS/abs@.nsf/DetailsPage/4839.02014-15?OpenDocument
9. Willis, E., Reynolds, L., Keleher, H.: Understanding the Australian Health System, 2nd edn. Elsevier, Amsterdam (2014)
10. Department of Health and Ageing: The readiness of Australian General Practitioners for the eHealth record (2011)
11. Australia Digital Health Agency: My health record statistics as at 25 February 2018 (2018). https://myhealthrecord.gov.au/internet/mhr/publishing.nsf/Content/news-002
12. Koh, T.: New PIP requirement betrays blinkered approach. Medicus 56(1), 33 (2016). (in English)
13. Wade, T.N., Annapurna: GP change management strategy: engagement with general practice. HealthConnect SA, Adelaide (2006). https://nla.gov.au/nla.cat-vn3944689
14. Raza Khan, U., Zia, T.: Literature review about MyHR adoption in general practices. In: Presented at the 2017 Higher Degree Research Symposium, Wagga, NSW, Book of Short Papers (2017)
15. Raza Khan, U., Zia, T., Perera, K., Pearce, C.: The my health record (MyHR) adoption in general practices: literature review and future research direction (2018). Submitted to ITMR
16. Muhammad, I., Teoh, S.Y., Wickramasinghe, N.: Why using actor network theory (ANT) can help to understand the personally controlled electronic health record (PCEHR) in Australia. Int. J. Act. Netw. Theory Technol. Innov. (IJANTTI) 4(2), 44–60 (2012)
17. Kerai, P., Wood, P., Martin, M.: A pilot study on the views of elderly regional Australians of personally controlled electronic health records. Int. J. Med. Inform. Prespectives Eval. 83(3), 201–209 (2014)
18. Spiranovic, C., Matthews, A., Scanlan, J., Kirkby, K.C.: Personally controlled electronic health records in Australia: challenges in communication of mental health information. Adv. Ment. Health 12(2), 147–153 (2014). (in English)
19. van Dooren, K., Lennox, N., Stewart, M.: Improving access to electronic health records for people with intellectual disability: a qualitative study. Aust. J. Prim. Health Prespectives Eval. 19(4), 336–342 (2013)

20. Raza Khan, U.: Study of eHealth in Australia and its adoption in Regional Victoria (Australia). MSc Business Strategic and Information Systems, Business School, University of Hertfordshire (2013)

21. Lehnbom, E., McLachlan, A., Brien, J.-A.: A qualitative study of Australians' opinions about personally controlled electronic health records. Stud. Health Technol. Inform. Prespectives Eval. **178**, 105–110 (2012)

22. Lehnbom, E.C., Brien, J.E., McLachlan, A.J.: Knowledge and attitudes regarding the personally controlled electronic health record: an Australian national survey. Intern. Med. J. Prespectives Eval. **44**(4), 406–409 (2014)

23. Mooranian, A., Emmerton, L., Hattingh, L.: The introduction of the national e-health record into Australian community pharmacy practice: pharmacists' perceptions. Int. J. Pharm. Pract. Prespectives Eval. **21**(6), 405–412 (2013)

24. Quinlivan, J.A., Lyons, S., Petersen, R.W.: Attitudes of pregnant women towards personally controlled electronic, hospital-held, and patient-held medical record systems: a survey study. Telemed. E-Health Prespectives Eval. **20**(9), 810–815 (2014)

25. Lehnbom, E.C., Douglas, H.E., Makeham, M.A.B.: Positive beliefs and privacy concerns shape the future for the Personally Controlled Electronic Health Record. Intern. Med. J. Framew. Eval **46**(1), 108–111 (2016)

26. Srur, B.L., Drew, S.: Challenges in designing a successful e-health system for Australia. In: International Symposium on Information Technology in Medicine and Education (ITME), vol. 1, pp. 480–484 (2012)

27. Xu, J., Gao, X., Sorwar, G., Croll, P.: Current Status, Challenges, and Outlook of E-Health Record Systems in Australia. In: Sun, F., Li, T., Li, H. (eds.) Knowledge Engineering and Management. AISC, vol. 214, pp. 683–692. Springer, Heidelberg (2014). https://doi.org/10. 1007/978-3-642-37832-4_62

28. Najaftorkaman, M., Ghapanchi, A.H., Talaei-Khoei, A.: Effectiveness of a personally controlled electronic health record intervention in older adults with chronic disease. In: Presented at the 26th Australasian Conference on Information Systems, Adelaide (2015). https://acis2015.unisa.edu.au/wp-content/uploads/2015/11/ACIS_2015_paper_14.pdf

29. Almond, H., Cummings, E., Turner, P.: Avoiding failure for Australia's digital health record: the findings from a rural e-health participatory research project. In: Digital Health Innovation for Consumers, Clinicians, Connectivity and Community: Selected Papers from the 24th Australian National Health Informatics Conference (HIC 2016), vol. 227, p. 8. IOS Press (2016)

30. Pearce, C., Bartlett, J., McLeod, A., Eustace, P., Amos, R., Shearer, M.: Effectiveness of local support for the adoption of a national programme-a descriptive study. Inform. Prim. Care Prespectives Eval. **21**(4), 171–178 (2014)

31. Hemsley, et al.: The personally controlled electronic health record (PCEHR) for adults with severe communication impairments: findings of pilot research. Stud. Health Technol. Inform. Prespectives Eval. **214**, 100–106 (2015)

32. Gajanayake, R., Sahama, T., Iannella, R.: E-health in Australia and elsewhere: a comparison and lessons for the near future. Stud. Health Technol. Inform. **188**, 26–32 (2013)

33. Knight, A.W., Szucs, C., Dhillon, M., Lembke, T., Mitchell, C.: The eCollaborative: using a quality improvement collaborative to implement the National eHealth Record System in Australian primary care practices. Int. J. Qual. Health Care Framew. Eval. **26**(4), 411–417 (2014)

34. Spriggs, M., Arnold, M.V., Pearce, C.M., Fry, C.: Ethical questions must be considered for electronic health records. J. Med. Eth. **38**(9), 535–539 (2012)

35. DoH: Digital health data (2018). http://www.health.gov.au/internet/main/publishing.nsf/ Content/PHN-Digital_Health

Extraction of Semantic Relations from Medical Literature Based on Semantic Predicates and SVM

Xiaoli Zhao[1]($\boxtimes$), Shaofu Lin[1], and Zhisheng Huang[2]

[1] College of Software, Beijing University of Technology, Beijing, China
`zhaoxiaoli@emails.bjut.edu.cn`, `linshaofu@bjut.edu.cn`
[2] Department of Computer Science,
VU University Amsterdam, Amsterdam, The Netherlands
`huang@cs.vu.nl`

Abstract. The relationship of biomedical entity is the cornerstone of acquiring biomedical knowledge. It is of great significance to the construction of related databases in the biomedical field and the management of medical literature. How to quickly and accurately extract the required relationships of biomedical entity from massive unstructured literature is an important research. In order to improve accuracy, we use support vector machine (SVM) which is a machine learning algorithm based on feature vectors to extract relationships of entities. We extract the five main relationships in medical literature, including ISA, PART_OF, CAUSES, TREATS and DIAGNOSES. First of all, related topics are used to search medical literature from PubMed database, such as disease-drug, cause-disease. These documents are used as experimental data and then processed to form a corpus. In selection of features, the method of information gain is used to select the influential entities' own features and entities' context features. On this basis, semantic predicates are added as a feature to improve accuracy. The experimental results show that the accuracy of extraction is increased by 5%–10%. In the end, Resource Description Framework (RDF) is used to store extracted relationships from the corresponding documents, and it provides support for the subsequent retrieval of related documents.

Keywords: Relation extraction · Semantic technology · SVM
Multi-classification · RDF

1 Introduction

A large number of biomedical literatures are the valuable results of medical research. Excavating biomedical literature in depth can not only fully improve the utilization rate of medical literature, but also continuously promote the development of medicine [1]. The deep mining of the medical literature through natural language processing technology has received extensive attention in domestic and abroad. We mainly use the natural language technology to carry on relational extraction from the medical literature. At present, the extraction of semantic relation mainly focuses on the extraction of therapeutic relationships, including relationships and mutation relationships etc. It is of

© Springer Nature Switzerland AG 2018
S. Siuly et al. (Eds.): HIS 2018, LNCS 11148, pp. 17–24, 2018.
https://doi.org/10.1007/978-3-030-01078-2_2

great significance for building domain knowledge maps, knowledge bases and clinical decision support systems [2].

However, the method of feature-based extraction lacks optimization in selection of features, and a large number of features lead to low efficiency of experiment. Due to the loss of some important features, the accuracy of the experiment is reduced. This study improves the accuracy of extraction by optimizing features and adding new features.

The rest of this paper is organized as follows. Section 2 gives an overview of related works. Section 3 introduces research methods. Section 4 illustrates experimental procedure. Section 5 makes an analysis of the experimental results. The last section includes conclusions and future work.

2   Related Work

The research on the extraction of semantic relations in biomedical literature has been developed in domestic and abroad for many years. As an important application in the biomedical field, natural language processing and machine learning, and it has gained extensive attention from researchers of related fields. At present, the extracted methods of relationships are mainly divided into knowledge-based and machine learning-based.

Knowledge-based extraction of relationships mainly relies on medical knowledge resources and combines with co-occurrence analysis, symbolic natural language processing, and manual summary rules [2]. Hassan [3] in 2015 years used the dependency graph to automatically learn the syntactic pattern of relational extraction, and selected the best mode according to accuracy and specificity. Finally, they used this model to extract the relationships of disease-symptom in the new text, and the accuracy was 55.65%. Although knowledge-based extraction can achieve better results in a particular field, but it needs to spend a lot of time, energy and poor portability.

Methods of extraction based on Machine-learning include feature vectors and kernel. Zheng [4] in 2016 represented words of different contexts and distances as vectors for extracting drug-drug interactions and the accuracy was 68.4%. Bi Haibin [5] in 2012 used the SVM algorithm and proposed a construction method of semantic feature based on CNKI. Finally, the accuracy reached 75%. Although these experiments have achieved good results, there is a lack of optimization in feature selection.

The SVM algorithm is used to extract the relationships in this paper. It adopts not only the common features in previous studies, but also selects influential features through information gain to improve the efficiency of the experiment. Considering that semantic predicates play a very important role in the recognition of semantic relationships, we propose to add semantic predicates as a new feature.

3   Method

3.1   Selection of Relationships

It is an important step for this study to select reasonable extracted relationships. Semantic Medline proposes 58 typical semantic relationships [6] such as ISA,

LOCATION_OF, PART OF, USES, CAUSES, TREATS, DIAGNOSES and so on. Because of the large number of relationships, we first select five typical relationships to extract, namely, ISA, PART_OF, CAUSES, TREATS, DIAGNOSES. The remaining relationships will be further expanded according to the experimental results in the future.

3.2 Selection of Features

We transform relational extraction into a multi-classification problem, and use SVM based on feature vector to extract. Therefore, the better selection of features has a great impact on the efficiency of the experiment. Then the selected features are extracted from the experimental data and mapped into the feature vector to do the experiment. Considering that the number of extracted features is relatively large and the dimension of the feature vector is too high, we adopt the method of information gain (IG) to filter the features, Finally we select the features that have a relatively large impact on extraction, mainly including the entity's own features and the entity's context features

From the perspective of linguistics, the entities are nouns basically. Its position and role in the sentence fulfill certain statistical laws [7]. Therefore, the feature of the entity itself has important significance to the extraction of the entity's relationship. The entity's own features selected in this paper are as follows:

(1) The location of the entity: The location of the entity refers to the location of the two entities in the sentence
(2) Entity distance: the distance between two entities
(3) Entity Type: Concept of Entity Ownership

From the perspective of the part-of-speech tagging, the part-of-speech of each component in the sentence is also relatively fixed [7]. Therefore, the feature of the entity's context has a certain guiding effect on the extraction of the relationship of the entities. At the same time, in order to obtain better semantic expression capabilities, We select the parts of speech and word vector features as the lexical features. entity's context features are as follows:

(1) Word items between two entities
(2) The first two word terms of the first entity
(3) Word terms after the second entity

3.3 Semantic Predicate Features

The description of the biomedical relationships is mainly based on some predicates that can reflect the semantic relationship in the sentence. Using these predicates to extract the relationship can accurately show the rules of the relation between the entities in the complex sentences, and have a better effect in judging the relationship of entities [8]. We collect the common semantic predicates in medical literature, and refer to the related semantic predicates of UMLS.

For example, Blood-retinal barrier (BRB) breakdown and vascular leakage is the leading cause of blindness of diabetic retinopathy (DR). The sentence includes two

Table 1. Features and corresponding values of the example

Features	Value of features
PMID	29402864
Location of the first entity	1
Location of the second entity	12
The distance between entities	10
The category of first entity	Symptom
The category of second entity	Disease
Two word items before the first entity	0
Two word items after second entities	0
Word items between entities	Cause blindness and so on
Semantic predicate features	Cause

entities, namely, BRB and DR, and they belong to the symptom and disease respectively. Each value of features are as follows (Table 1):

3.4 Support Vector Machine (SVM)

The purpose of the support vector machine algorithm is to find a hyperplane. The hyperplane can separate the data in the training set, and the distance from the category boundary to the hyperplane is the largest. Therefore, the algorithm is also called the maximum edge algorithm, which has strong adaptability and high accuracy. In addition, the support vector machine algorithm is not limited by the theory that the sample tends to infinity, so the automatic classification has a high accuracy in small samples [9, 10]. Therefore, this research transforms relational extraction into a multi-classification problem and uses SVM algorithm to extract relationships.

4 Experimental Procedure

4.1 Sources of Data

We mainly extract the relationship of entities from the English medical literature. The experimental data is from medical literature in the PubMed database. Retrieving related medical literature by keywords such as "depressive disorder"[MeSHTerms], "therapy" [Subheading] "diabetes mellitus"[MeSHTerms],"therapy"[Subheading], etc. Finally, about 150 abstracts were collected as experimental data. After the pretreatment, 300 sentences contained entities were used as experimental data (Fig. 1).

4.2 Normalization of Experiment Corpus

Considering the redundancy and non-standard features of data in medical literature, the first step is to preprocess the abstract. The ICTCLAS2016 participle system is used to preprocess the data in clauses, participle, and part of speech tagging. Finally, we use java programs to select sentences containing related entities as experimental corpus.

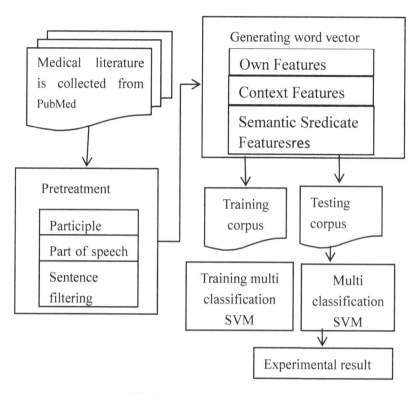

Fig. 1. Experimental flow chart

In order to illustrate the extracted relation belongs to that document, we label the PMID as a feature at the beginning of the sentence.

4.3 Construction of Feature Vector

In the experiment, we need to construct the feature vector as the input of the algorithm. According to the selected features in 3.1, we need to digitize each feature separately. The position and distance of the entity's own features are the corresponding values directly. The value of each category is based on the quantity. The context features of entities include part of speech and word vectors, and all the parts of speech are numbered as the value of part of speech. We uses the Word2Vec open source tool to generate word vectors [11, 12], which uses a deep-dense dense vector (Word Embedding) instead of the One-Hot vector used in traditional methods [13]. It can be better used as a word representation of entity context features (Table 2).

4.4 Training Model

We used LIBSVM (A Library for Support Vector Machines integration tool) [14] to extract relation of entities. Firstly we use function with parameters optimized to get the

Table 2. Feature vector of the example

Features	Value of Features
PMID	29402864
Location of the first entity	1
Location of the second entity	12
The distance between entities	10
The category of first entity	3
The category of second entity	1
Two word items before the first entity	0
Two word items after second entities	0
Word items between entities	0.62 0.12 …
Semantic predicate features	4

optimized parameters c = 0.73, g = 0.03, and then, we began to train the model and test the data.

5 Results and Analysis

5.1 Standard of Evaluation

P(Accuracy), R(recall), and F(F-measure) are used as evaluation criteria in this experiment. They are defined as follows:

$$P = T/E$$

$$R = T/N$$

$$F = 2 * P * R/(P + R)$$

Where T is the number of instances that are correctly classified for a certain class, N is the actual total number of a category in the tested data, and E is the classifiers predict the total number of a category.

5.2 Experimental Results

In this study, information gain is used to optimize the features. on this basis, we propose to add semantic predicates as new features. By comparing the experimental results, we find that adding semantic predicates can improve the accuracy of extraction. It also provides a new extension of feature selection in the future (Table 3).

5.3 Storage of Results

In this paper, the triples (entity, relationship, entity) of extracted relationship are stored in the form of RDF, so as to facilitate the retrieval of related documents in the future [15].

Table 3. Experimental result

Relationships features	Own features context features			Own features context features semantic predicate features		
	P	R	F	P	R	F
ISA	0.75	0.64	0.69	0.79	0.68	0.73
PART_OF	0.62	0.54	0.57	0.76	0.65	0.70
CAUSES	0.78	0.76	0.77	0.79	0.76	0.77
TREATS	0.64	0.63	0.64	0.74	0.62	0.67
DIAGNOSES	0.77	0.51	0.61	0.78	0.60	0.68

The PMID of related literature is defined in RDF, and five main relationships are set as attributes. Because the unique identifier PMID of the medical document has been retained as a feature in the sentence when the experimental data is preprocessed, the relationship extracted from the corresponding PMID may be added as an attribute value, and finally saved in the form of RDF.

6 Conclusion and Future Work

SVM algorithm based on the feature vector was used to extract the among five relationships of entities from the biomedical literature, such as disease-drug, etiology-disease, etc. Although the semantic predicate feature is added to improve the accuracy of extraction, but the related entities and semantic predicates were extracted from the experimental data, so it had certain limitations. Therefore, the next study can use semi-supervised learning to extract and making full use of existing medical knowledge makes the result more universal.

References

1. Yang, Z.: Research of Text Mining Technology in Biomedical Field. Dalian University of Technology, Dalian (2008)
2. Li, F., Liu, S., Liu, Z.: A review of semantic relation extraction methods in biomedicine. Libr. Forum **6**, 61–69 (2017)
3. Hassan, M., Makkaoui, O., Coulet, A., et al.: Extracting disease-symptom relationships by learning syntactic patterns from dependency graphs. In: Proceedings of the 2015 Workshop on Biomedical Natural Language Processing (BioNLP 2015), pp. 71–80 (2015)
4. Zheng, W., Lin, H., Zhao, Z., et al.: A graph kernel based on context vectors for extracting drug–drug interactions. J Biomed Inform. **61**, 34–43 (2016)
5. Bi, H., et al.: The extraction of Chinese entity's relation based on semantic and SVM. In: National Conference on Information Storage Technology (2012)

6. Kilicoglu, H., Fiszman, M., Rodriguez, A., Shin, D.: AM ripple. Semantic MEDLINE: a web application for managing the results of PubMed searches. In: Proceedings of Smbm, pp. 69–76 (2008)
7. Fang, L.: Research on Two Stage Named Entity Recognition of Chinese Micro-Blog Based on CRF. Xihua University, Chengdu (2015)
8. Xiu Yan, W., et al.: Extracting semantic relations between biomedical entities by hybrid method. Mod. Library Inf. Technol. 29(3), 77–82 (2013)
9. Cristianini, N., Shawe-Taylor, J., Li, G., Wang, M., Zeng, H.J.: Introduction of Support Vector Machine. Publishing House of Electronics Industry, Beijing (2004)
10. Hang, Li: Statistical Machine Learning. Tsinghua University Press, Beijing (2012)
11. Zhang, Y., Xu, J., Chen, H., et al.: Chemical named entity recognition in patents by domain knowledge and unsupervised feature learning. J. Biol. Databases Curation (2016)
12. He, H.: Research of Word Representations on Biomedical Named Entity Recognition. Dalian University of Technology, Dalian (2015)
13. Collobert, R., Weston, J., Bottou, L., et al.: Natural language processing (almost) fromscratch. J. Mach. Learn. Res. 12, 2493–2537 (2011)
14. LIBSVM: A library for support vector machines [CP/DK]. https://www.csie.ntu.edu.tw
15. Gao, X.: The Construction of Entity Relationship Model Based on RDF(S) Resource Query. Jilin University, Changchun (2017)

Decision Making for Traditional Chinese Medicine Based on Fuzzy Cognitive Map

Daniel Lee[1,2](✉), Huai Liu[1] (iD), Jia Rong[1], Hong Xu[1],
and Yuan Miao[1]

[1] College of Engineering and Science, Victoria University, Melbourne, Australia
daniel.lee@chineseharmony.com.au,
{huai.liu,jia.rong,hong.xu,yuan.miao}@vu.edu.au
[2] Harmony Chinese Medicine Osteopathy and Acupuncture,
Kew, VIC 3101, Australia

Abstract. One fundamental concept in Traditional Chinese Medicine (TCM) is to consider the human body as a whole, inside which the functions of various body organs are inseparable in terms of mutual coordination as well as the physiological and pathological influences among one another. It is believed in TCM that the human body is also integrated with the living environment through causal relationships. Similar to the basic rationale of TCM, Fuzzy Cognitive Mapping (FCM) is a technique that considers knowledge as a whole. It attempts to simulate normal human reasoning and human decision-making processes. It is thus natural to apply FCM to represent knowledge and experience in TCM treatments. In this paper, we propose to use an FCM-based approach to support decision making for TCM. The approach is evaluated through a case study based on the TCM treatment of common cold. It is clearly shown that the FCM-based approach can provide improvements in the efficiency and precision of decision making for TCM doctors.

Keywords: Traditional Chinese Medicine · Fuzzy Cognitive Map
Decision making

1 Introduction

Traditional Chinese Medicine (TCM) has been popularly used in China for thousands of years. One fundamental rationale behind TCM is the belief that man and the universe are part of a whole unit. The relationship between humans and the universe is a dynamic causal correspondence. However, individual's adaptability and response to the natural environment are distinct, and the causal relationships behind these responses are different accordingly. It is believed in TCM that the relationships among human viscera are dynamically complicated in several distinct flavours. These flavours include independent, dependent, interdependent, co-dependent and counter-dependent types.

TCM practitioners make use of a so-called holistic approach as dialectics of aetiology and pathogenesis of TCM diagnostics. In combination with the information of patient's medical history, living environment, type of work and lifestyle, physical examinations are conducted via four major diagnostic methods: observation;

© Springer Nature Switzerland AG 2018
S. Siuly et al. (Eds.): HIS 2018, LNCS 11148, pp. 25–36, 2018.
https://doi.org/10.1007/978-3-030-01078-2_3

auscultation and olfaction; interrogation; and, pulse feeling and palpation. These methods can reflect messages for the pathological and physiological disharmony of a patient. Nevertheless, the accuracy and efficiency in diagnosis and decision making significantly rely on the individual TCM practitioner's knowledge and experience. Medical decision making is a complex procedure, evaluating a variety of causal factors and suggesting a diagnosis and decision. Computer-aided systems have been used to aid doctors in making patients' diagnosis and medical decision for decades. However, due to the complexity of TCM, computer-aided decision making has not yet been successful.

Fuzzy Cognitive Mapping (FCM) is a soft computing technique that follows a reasoning approach similar to human reasoning and human decision-making process. FCM has two major functions: one is to reason about the causal factors involved in prediction; and the other is to analyse the results from the causation. FCM can be a powerful tool to support decision making as the experience of experts and information from historical data can be combined and contribute to form the maps representing the knowledge [1–3].

A number of studies have been conducted to apply FCM into medical decision making, where FCM helps analyse the views and events that are carried on a medical subject with qualitative and quantitative ways. For example, FCM has been used in medical diagnosis, long-term prediction of diseases, disease risk assessment and disease management [4].

Similar to FCM, TCM also aims at finding the causal relationships among various factors to support decision making. It is thus natural to make use of the FCM technique to improve the accuracy and efficiency of TCM diagnosis. In this paper, we investigate the application of FCM into the decision making of TCM. We have conducted a case study based on treatments of common cold to demonstrate the applicability and effectiveness of the FCM-based decision making for TCM. Our results clearly show that the FCM can help make the correct decisions for the diagnosis and the corresponding treatment approaches.

The rest of the paper is structured as follows. In Sects. 2 and 3, we introduce the background information of TCM and FCM, respectively. In Sect. 4, we illustrate how to use FCM in the context of TCM based on a simple example. In Sect. 5, we report the case study for evaluating FCM's applicability in the decision making of TCM. In Sect. 6, we discuss the related work. Finally, we conclude the paper in Sect. 7.

2 Traditional Chinese Medicine

TCM is an ancient practice currently used by millions of people all over the world. The core of TCM is that the individual's microcosm is viewed as an integral part of nature's macrocosmos. Diagnosis in TCM may appear to be simply a grouping of symptoms and signs named as patterns of disharmony. Thus, the treatment strategy is to match the conclusion to the diagnostic pattern. For example, common cold has many patterns in TCM. The most common patterns fall under the categories of wind-cold and wind-heat. External symptoms of wind-cold may change very rapidly, therefore treatment strategies require adaptability over the course of the illness. The wind-cold pattern commonly presents the following symptoms and signs: fever, shivering, inability to get warm, sinus congestion with clear coloured mucus, cough with clear coloured phlegm, stiff nape and shoulders/upper back, occipital headache. A slower than normal pulse can be felt by the TCM practitioner from the surface of the skin (floating pulse). Diaphoretic (sweating) herbal therapy is especially helpful in this condition, which can warm the body internally and expel the cold pathogen out by sweating.

The very early stages of the wind-cold pattern can be treated effectively with a remedy of rice congee cooked with the bulb of spring onion and fresh ginger. In the case of advanced conditions, TCM practitioners will use a range of therapies, depending on the combination of symptoms.

When the influence of wind combines with heat, fever is more pronounced and the pulse is faster than normal. Sore throat is present as well as headache and irritability. If there is a cough, it is usually dry or non-productive, with occasional expectoration of yellow mucus at the early stage. Honey suckle flower, chrysanthemum and mulberry leaf tea can release the symptoms.

When treating cold or flu symptoms due to wind-heat, the results are always more effective if the treatment begins at the earliest possible stage of the illness. It is important to get adequate rest, minimize stress and drink soup and fresh juices. Sweets, tonics and spicy food may cause a rapid progression in the severity of the illness since they tend to feed the pathogen.

The distinction between building long-term immunity and fighting off an acute illness is an important idea within TCM. While tonic herbs may need to be taken long term, it is important to discontinue their use during an initial stage of cold or flu. Then, after the pathogen has been expelled from the body, the intake of tonic herbs can be resumed to build up strength and vitality over the long-term. For example, the individual who has weak general wellbeing (Qi deficiency) and often repeatedly catches common cold can take ginseng as a tonic to strengthen anti-pathogen vitality and resistance to cold, but should discontinue use once a cold is present.

If a person's resistance to disease is weak (a Qi deficiency) the person would not be able to recover from a cold easily, then a small dosage of ginseng or other Qi tonifying herbs combined with other herbs for expelling exogenous pathogens would be prescribed by a TCM practitioner.

Qi is the essential energy in the body and relates to the physiological functions of viscera and meridians. It is a vital energy which can be interpreted as the "life energy; life force" [5].

3   Fuzzy Cognitive Mapping

Fuzzy Cognitive Mapping (FCM) is a soft computing technique which can mimic the human reasoning process. Uncertain causal knowledge is stored in a map that is a fuzzy signed diagram with feedback. Unlike data driven models, FCM maps are built on human expertise. It represents and models human knowledge and expertise in decision making. FCM allows loops that can model widely ranging feedback. It is not a rigid model and allows multiple experts to contribute their knowledge without the need of compromise to maintain a certain structure (e.g., the tree structure in classic logic) [1–4, 6–10].

FCM can be represented as a signed fuzzy weighted graph with closed loops. It consisted of nodes and directed arcs connecting between them. FCM nodes represent variable phenomena or fuzzy sets. An FCM node nonlinearly transforms weighted summed inputs into numerical output, again in analogy to a dynamical system model neuron. FCM resonant states are limit cycles, or time-varying patterns. Figure 1 shows an example of FCM map. Each node in the map represents a concept (represented by V_i, where $i = 1, 2 \ldots$) in the problem demand. The interrelation between concepts is given by strength values (e.g., weight W_{12}) which reflect the degree of causal influence. The weights strongly incorporate the available knowledge and expertise in the field. The inference proceeds by nonlinear spreading activation.

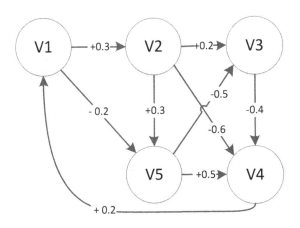

V1: Cancer Therapy, Type I, II, or III
V2: Cancer Stage
V3: Pain
V4: Life Performance KPS %
V5: Response to Therapy

Fig. 1. An example of FCM map

The weights strongly incorporate the available knowledge and expertise in the field. Normally, FCM weights can be determined by the following two methods:

- *From experts*: This is a typical approach. It appears to be a rough estimation at the start point but can be rather effective and accurate through continuous adjustments. For example, in the context of medicine, as doctors can view the whole process of the inference, they can thus easily see the inappropriate value of weights and make adjustments. Thus, the weights can be quite accurate after a few rounds of adjustment.

- *From data*: This is similar to any data approach for coefficient modelling. This will need sufficient data and multivariable analysis. In our study, we mainly focus on the method from experts, while the data-based weight modelling after initial knowledge structure of FCM is the next step of the study.

As discussed above, a strong alignment can be observed between the rationales of FCM and TCM. They both look at the causal relationships among various factors to guide reasoning and decision making. Therefore, it is interesting to see whether and to what extent FCM can be used in the computer-aided decision making for TCM, particularly aiming at improving the accuracy and efficiency of TCM diagnosis and treatment.

4 Illustration

In this section, we illustrate how to draw an FCM map for the decision making in TCM diagnosis and treatment, based on a syndrome called wind-cold. It mainly happens when an individual is invaded by exogenous pathogenic factors of wind and cold. It may be more prevalent in winter, or cold windy days, or in cold environments such as air-conditioned rooms. The clinical manifestations can be sneezing, headache, chills, runny nose, nasal congestion, cough, thin and clear sputum, muscle aches, absence of fever or low fever, thin white tongue coating, floating or floating tight pulse.

Based on the above knowledge from one of our authors, we built the FCM map as shown in Fig. 2. In the map, the concept "Wind Cold" represents the symptoms of wind-cold.

The treatment principle is to expel exogenous pathogens with characteristic warm herbs to dispel internal cold and promote lung function. The treatment is represented as "Treatment-WC0" and can be applied to address the fundamental symptoms. "Jing Fang Bai Du San formula" modification can be used as a basic prescription.

A patient may develop extra symptoms such as fever with shivering and lack of sweating represented by "Symptom-WC1"; excessive cough with abundant clear color phlegm represented by "Symptom-WC2"; severe headache represented by "Symptom-WC3"; rigid stiffness of nape and upper back represented by "Symptom-WC4"; and nausea represented by "Symptom-WC5".

For these extra symptoms, different additional treatments can be applied, by adding Ma Huang (Herba Ephedrae) and Gui Zhi (Ramulus Cinnamomi) to expel internal cold represented by "Treatment-WC1"; adding Xing Ren (Semen Armeniacae) and Zhe Bei Mu (Bulbus Fritillariae Thunbergii) to expel phlegm represented by "Treatment-WC2"; adding Bai Zhi (Radix Angelicae Dahuricae) to dispel wind pathogen and relieve headache represented by "Treatment-WC3"; adding Ge Gen (Radix Puerariae) to relieve tightness of muscles and relieve pain represented by "Treatment-WC4"; and adding "Xiang Shu San formula" represented by "Treatment-WC5". The weights among these concepts are provided by the expert.

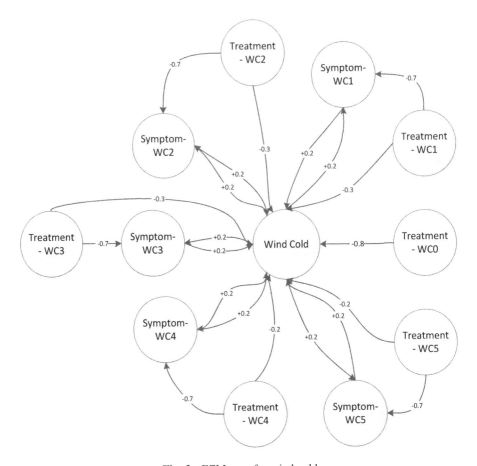

Fig. 2. FCM map for wind cold

5 Case Study

5.1 Objects

In this study, we evaluate the applicability of FCM in TCM based on common cold symptoms. In TCM, the common cold can be classified into different types such as wind-cold, wind-heat, and summer-heat with dampness. The deficiency types of cold are subdivided as Qi Deficiency (low energy); Blood Deficiency (poor blood supplement); Yang Deficiency (cold or hypo-activity type); Yin Deficiency (dry/false heat type).

Generally, a healthy person may have severe symptoms and can get recovered quickly if he or she catches a common cold from wind-cold; wind-heat; or summer-heat with dampness pathogen. Nevertheless, when a person who is under deficiency condition invaded by wind-cold pathogen, it can take much longer to get recovered.

During the treatment, it is very likely that the patient's disease will be converted into a different syndrome as well. For example, when a Qi deficient person catches a wind-cold, it can transfer from cold syndrome to heat that changes the symptoms accordingly as well. For such a case, the treatment principle is to improve the Qi deficiency and to relieve the symptoms of the cold.

If the symptoms of a wind-cold pathogen do not get treated and recovered in time, the cold patterned symptoms could then generate deficient heat and to be transformed to heat patterns, such as thirst and dry mouth and a desire to drink cold water; yellow thick phlegm; pharyngeal pain and other symptoms. The recurrence of cold can worsen the patient's Qi strength and can lead to recurrence of the cold as well. Common cold can also transmit issues such as palpitation and edema.

5.2 Experimental Results

We drew the FCM maps for wind-cold, wind-heat cold, summer-dampness cold, Qi-deficiency cold, blood-deficiency cold, Yang-deficiency cold, and Yin-deficiency cold. The map for wind-cold is already given in Fig. 2. Maps for wind-heat cold and the Qi-deficiency (low energy) cold patterns are shown in Figs. 3 and 4, respectively.

The wind-heat cold case shows how these maps help doctors make decisions on treatment. The primary symptoms of wind-heat cold include fever and aversion to wind, headache, nasal congestion with thick yellow discharge, cough with yellow phlegm, thirst and dry mouth, swollen pharynx, sore and red edge of the tongue, thin yellow coating on the tongue, rapid floating pulse. The fundamental treating principle (represented by "Treatment–WH0" in Fig. 3) is to use cold characteristic herbs to cool down the body and to expel the exogenous pathogens, namely, a basic prescription of "Yin Qiao San formula". The individual's symptoms can be variously distinct according the progress of the disease. In Fig. 3, "Symptom–WH1" represents severe sinus blockage, which can be treated by adding Shi Chang Pu (Rhizoma Acori Tatarinowii), Cang Er Zi (Fructus Xanthii), Xin Yi (Flos Magnoliae Lilliflorae) and Bai Zhi (Angelica Dahurica) to clear the sinus passage and relieve headache by dispelling pathogenic wind factors ("Treatment–WH1"). "Symptom–WH2" denotes severe headache, treated by adding Sang Ye (Folium Mori), Ju Hua (Flos Chrysanthemi) and Man Jing Zi (Fructus Viticis) to expel heat and for enforcing the circulations of the meridians around the head for headache relief ("Treatment–WH2"). "Symptom–WH3" represents severe swollen and sore throat, treated by adding Xuan Shen (Radix Scro-phulariae), Ma Bo (Lasiosphera/Calvatia) and Ban Lan Gen (Radix Isatidis) as anti-pyretic and detoxifying remedies to relieve sore throat ("Treatment–WH3"). "Symptom–WH4" represents excessive thirst and dry mouth, treated by adding Tian Hua Fen (Trichosanthes kirilowii), Lu Gen (Rhizoma Phragmitis) and Zhi Mu (Rhi-zoma Anemarrhenae) to clear heat and improve saliva production to relieve thirst ("Treatment–WH4"). "Symptom–WH5" denotes high fever, treated by adding Huang Qin (Radix Scutellariae), Shi Gao (Gypsum Fibrosum) and Da Qing Ye (Folium Isa-tidis) to clear internal heat for getting rid of fever ("Treatment–WH5"). "Symptom–WH6" represents cough with thick yellow phlegm, which can be treated by adding

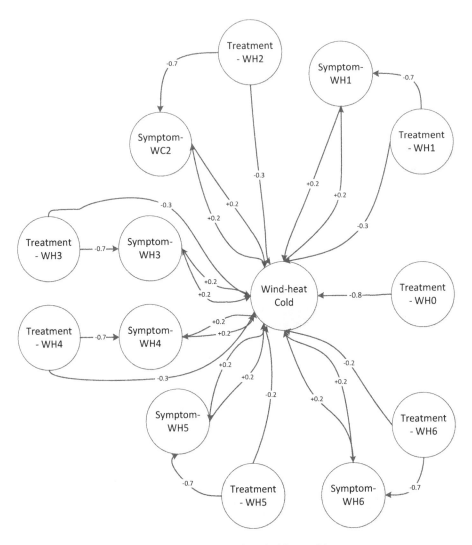

Fig. 3. FCM map for wind-heat cold

Huang Qin (Radix Scutellariae), Zhi Mu (Rhizoma Anemarrhenae), Zhe Bei Mu (Bulbus Fritillariae Thunbergii), Xing Ren (Semen Armeniacae) and Gua Lou Ren (Trichosanthis Semen) to expel phlegm for clearing lung turbidity ("Treatment–WH6").

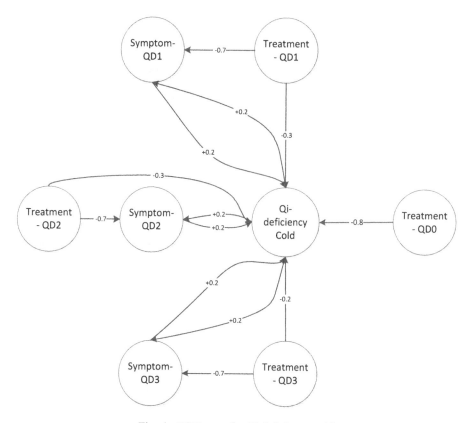

Fig. 4. FCM map for Qi-deficiency cold

6 Related Work

Some work has been done to investigate the efficiency of FCM to model the established knowledge for the specific application of breast cancer risk assessment. It was concluded that the proposed decision support approach has the capacity to accurately evaluate the breast cancer risk factors and to assess the overall risk grade, providing clinical oncologists with information for adjusting the patients' intervention procedure [11].

Another study at the Adyar cancer institute was focused on analysing the symptoms of breast cancer for 100 women between 26 and 65 years old by using FCM models. The models used expert opinions as the input. It was concluded that use of FCM model analysis can accurately evaluate the risk of breast cancer from the causal relationships of breast pain with other critical symptoms of nipple turning inward, redness, scarring, thickness of nipple/breast skin and abnormal discharge [11].

An enhanced version of the evolutionary learning approach of FCMs, involving consideration of a parameter that defines a long prediction horizon, was investigated for the prediction of prostate cancer. It was concluded that the fitness function of the enhanced learning algorithm enabled a better optimization of FCM for the task of long-term prediction of multivariate time series. The calculated prediction errors were small for the FCM-II due to the improved optimization of FCM that was accomplished using the approach. The proposed solution was validated in a pilot study using real medical data [12].

Another study on brain tumour concluded that the results of the proposed grading model present reasonably high accuracy and are comparable with existing algorithms such as decision trees and fuzzy decision trees. The main advantage of the proposed FCM grading model is the interpretability and transparency in the decision-making process, which makes it a convenient consulting tool in characterizing tumor aggressiveness for every day clinical practice [1]. Furthermore, the ability of the FCMs to model and structure accumulated knowledge and expertise might be an important contributor in enhancing the pathologists' consensus at the diagnostic level.

Medical Decision Making is a complex procedure – evaluating a variety of causal factors and arriving at a conclusive diagnosis and decision. Computer systems have been used in aiding doctors to make patients' diagnoses and medical decisions for many decades. In order to reduce doctors' work load in making accurate medical decisions, it is important to have a consistent system as a support. The system has to process and evaluate a high amount of data from multi-disciplinary sources such as patients' background information and records, doctors' physical examinations, laboratory tests, medical device examinations treatment results [13].

A study on FCM structures for Medical Decision Support Systems (MDSS) has concluded that soft computing techniques such as FCMs can be used as a consistent MDSS, achieving better solutions in diagnosis, treatment, prediction and so on. FCMs can be a powerful tool as the experience of many experts and knowledge from historical data can be combined and contribute to form the FCMs [13].

A study has been done on the modelling of medical knowledge and the behaviour of the system for decision support in urinary tract infection (UTI) diagnosis based on using FCMs implemented in a Semantic Web approach. This work establishes a decision support tool based on FCM formalism for UTI diagnosis by proposing the appropriate diagnosis for each individual case [14]. In a word, FCM is suitable for medical Decision Support Systems by helping analyse the views and events that are carried on a medical subject with qualitative and quantitative methods [4].

There do not exist Western medical laboratory tests or Western modern medical device examination reports to assist TCM practitioners in doing diagnostic decision-making. Nevertheless, within 10 to 20 min in an initial consultation, the TCM practitioner makes a diagnosis and decision for treatment.

The duty of a TCM practitioner is not only as medical practitioner of TCM but also to be an herbal medicine specialist. It is a very difficult task for a TCM practitioner to remember hundreds of Chinese herbs for safe and effective diagnostic decision-making within minutes. Nevertheless, diagnosis in TCM may appear to be simply a grouping of symptoms and signs, named as patterns of disharmony. Through clear differentiation among the patterns, the diagnosis is then concluded for decision making. For example, in this study, the common cold can be clearly differentiated into seven subclasses by patterns, each of which individually presents a syndrome. Once the data of diagnosis are filled into the FCM system, it will be computerised in analysis of the symptoms and classify into a TCM pattern. Hence, in TCM, it can be easy to do diagnose through FCM computing system by differentiation from the patterns for decision making support in clinical practice for TCM practitioners.

In TCM in the last decade there has been a tongue detecting device used to do tongue diagnosis, replacing the TCM practitioner's observation by taking photos of a patient's tongue for computer analysis. It was based on the Fuzzy C – Means Clustering algorithm for decision making in the diagnosis. Thus, it has proved that FCM can be used as clinical decision-making support system for TCM [15].

In recent decades TCM has been widely accepted as alternative medicine and many Western Integrative medicine practitioners have included TCM as part of their treatment approach. To improve the diagnostic accuracy of traditional Chinese medicine, improve the curative effect and ensure the patient's safety, the modernization of TCM with innovative technologies is necessary.

In this study, we propose an FCM-based approach to decision making in TCM. The approach is evaluated through a case study based on the TCM treatment of common cold. It is clearly shown that the FCM-based approach can provide efficient and precise decision making for TCM doctors. Therefore, it is demonstrated that FCM technology can help modernize TCM and make the related medical activities easier.

7 Conclusion

The TCM theoretical system is a large combination of interrelated theories. The theoretical system of TCM is based on ancient Chinese philosophical speculation and is more associated with the philosophy of intuitive thinking than mathematical models.

TCM is used in intuitive thinking models that are transformed from real things. The system of models of TCM may seem messy but after careful analysis it can be found that models of TCM can be classified according to different levels of consciousness. Models can take the following forms:

- perceptual forms, such as exterior, interior, cold and heat models
- reasonable forms, such as dynamic Qi circulation and meridian transmission model
- philosophical, such as the Yin and Yang model and the five elements model
- a mixture of intuition, sub-consciousness and philosophy, such as the unity of man and nature.

These different types of intuitive models are stored at the corresponding levels of consciousness. The interaction of consciousness hierarchy requires that they tend to be consistent, so that they each have a reasonable basis [16].

In this paper, we investigated the application of FCM in the decision making of TCM. Particularly, we have conducted a case study based on the treatments for common cold to demonstrate the applicability and effectiveness of the FCM-based decision making for TCM. The result of our experiment demonstrated that FCM can be used as a clinical decision-making support system and improve the diagnostic accuracy of TCM, improve the curative effect, ensure the patient's medication safety and help TCM practitioners' medical activities easier. However, there is a lot more work required for more comprehensive research to achieve further development of TCM modernization.

References

1. Papageorgiou, E.I., et al.: Brain tumor characterization using soft computing technique of fuzzy cognitive maps. Appl. Soft Comput. **8**, 820–828 (2008)
2. Subramanian, J., Karmegam, A., Papageorgiou, E., Papandrianos, N., Vasukie, A.: An integrated breast cancer risk assessment and management model based on fuzzy cognitive maps. Comput. Methods Prog. Biomed. **118**, 280–297 (2015)
3. Miao, Y.: Visualising fuzzy cognitive maps. In: WCCI 2012 IEEE World Congress on Computational Intelligence (2012)
4. Papageorgiou, E.I.: A new methodology for decisions in medical informatics using fuzzy cognitive maps based on fuzzy rule-extraction techniques. Appl. Soft Comput. **11**(1), 500–513 (2011)
5. Shen-nong TCM Basic Principles, Qi (Vital Energy) from a TCM Prospective. http://www.shen-nong.com/eng/principles/qi.html
6. Trendowski, M.: The promise of sonodynamic therapy: using ultrasound irradiation and chemotherapeutic agents as a treatment modality. Honors Capstone Project in Biolo, Renee Crown University Honors Program at Syracuse University (2014)
7. The Dove Clinic for Integrated Medicine Twyford & London Masters: PDT: PDT/SDT Study - 116 Patients (2009)
8. Miao, Y.: Fuzzy cognitive map for domain experts with no artificial intelligence expertise. In: Proceedings ICARCV, pp. 486–492 (2014)
9. Miao, Y.: Modelling dynamic causal relationship in fuzzy cognitive maps. In: Proceedings of International Conference on Fuzzy Systems, pp. 1013–1020 (2014)
10. Kosko, B.: Hidden patterns in combined and adaptive knowledge networks. Int. J. Approx. Reason. **2**(2), 377–393 (1998)
11. Bourgani, E., Stylios, C.D., Georgopoulos, V.C., Manis, G.: A study on the symptoms of breast cancer using fuzzy cognitive maps. In: 8th Conference of the European Society for Fuzzy Logic and Technology (2013)
12. Froelich, W., Papageorgiou, E.I., Samarinas, M., Skriapas, K.: Application of evolutionary fuzzy cognitive maps to the long-term prediction of prostate cancer. Appl. Soft Comput. **12**, 3810–3817 (2012)
13. Bourgani, E.A., Stylios, C.D., Georgopoulos, V.C., Manis, G.: A study on fuzzy cognitive map structures for medical decision support systems. In: 8th Conference of the European Society for Fuzzy Logic and Technology (2013)
14. Douali, N., Papageorgiou, E.I., De Roo, J., Cools, H., Jaulent, M.-C.: Clinical decision support system based on fuzzy cognitive maps. J. Comput. Sci. Syst. Biol. **8**, 112–120 (2015)
15. Jee, C.-C., Chiang, J.Y.: Automatic feature extraction and fuzzy analysis of sublingual veins. Taiwan Zhong Shan University (1999). http://hdl.handle.net/11296/5w2u4p
16. Wang, Z.-K.: To view the cognitive map in natural aspect - model reasoning and its methodological implications in TCM diagnosis (Chinese version). http://blog.sina.com.cn/s/blog_a6eb92f00102vz7k.html

Accelerometer-Based Physical Activity Patterns and Correlates of Depressive Symptoms

Xia Li[1(✉)], Patricia M. Kearney[2], and Anthony P. Fitzgerald[2]

[1] La Trobe University, Melbourne, VIC, Australia
lixia_new@163.com
[2] University College Cork, Cork, Ireland
{patricia.kearney, t.fitzgerald}@ucc.ie

Abstract. Background: A number of observational and intervention studies have investigated the relationship between physical activity and mental health; however, few studies evaluate the association between physical activity and depression in a population sample by using minute by minute data over one week from accelerometer. The purpose of this study is to explore the different physical activity patterns and the relationships between these patterns and depression symptoms based on minute by minute accelerometer assessed data. Methods: Data from the Mitchelstown cohort study were used. Taking consider of non-wear time and background information missing, 375 participants were included in this study. They all completed questionnaires and wore accelerometers for seven consecutive days. Questionnaire provided background information and Center for Epidemiological Studies Depression Scale (CES-D) score measurements, accelerometer output provided minute by minute physical activity data. Bivariate smoothing method was used to explore the interaction effect of depression score and other continuous background covariates to CES-D, multiple regression analysis was used to get the relationship between CES-D score and physical activity level. Results: Within Day Physical activity profile analysis showed that after 11:00 pm and before around 7:00 am, participants in moderate and moderate to severe depression groups are much active than the other two groups, but during the other day time, moderate to severe group is less active than the others. There were strong contrasts between depression groups regarding time-of day of peak per minute activity. Daily activity gets progressively lower for moderate to severe group since between 7 am and 8 am, and the cumulative activity is the lowest among these four groups. Bivariate relationship analysis also showed there were difference between male and female, different depression groups participants.

Keywords: Physical activity · Tri-axial · Accelerometer · Depression Bivariate smoothing

S. Siuly et al. (Eds.): HIS 2018, LNCS 11148, pp. 37–47, 2018.
https://doi.org/10.1007/978-3-030-01078-2_4

1 Introduction

Depression is a common mental disorder characterized by sadness, loss of interest or pleasure, feelings of guilt or low self-esteem, disturbed sleep or appetite, feelings of tiredness, and poor concentration. According to the World Health Organization (WHO 2012), more than 350 million people of all ages suffered from depression during 2012, and the World Mental Health Survey conducted in 17 countries found that on average about 1 in 20 people reported having an episode of depression in the previous year. By 2030 it is expected to be the largest contributor to disease burden (WHO 2008).

A number of observational and intervention studies have investigated the relationship between physical activity and mental health. Although findings have not been entirely consistent, many studies suggest that physical activity or exercise could reduce symptoms of mild to moderate depression (e.g. Babyak et al. 2000; Foley et al. 2008; Mota-Pereira et al. 2011). Some observational studies provided information on levels of physical activity (Thirlaway and Benton 1992; Paffenbarger et al. 1994; Hassmen et al. 2000; Brown et al. 2005; Wise et al. 2006), and concluded that both higher and lower levels of physical activity were associated with a decreased likelihood of depression. Some intervention studies clearly specified the frequency and duration of the training programs involved. These studies varied in terms of the frequency and intensity prescribed and some directly compared physical activity interventions of varying doses (Klein et al. 1985; Emery and Blumenthal 1988; Blumenthal et al. 1989; Moses et al. 1989; King et al. 1993; Brown et al. 1995; DiLorenzo et al. 1999).

In most of these studies, physical activity was assessed using measures such as the validated physical activity index (Young et al. 1995) and the long version of the International Physical Activity Questionnaire (IPAQ). These are all subjective measures, rely on a person recalling or remembering which activities they participated in, or recalling their perception of the intensity of the session. In some other studies, accelerometers were used to obtain the objective measures of physical activity, and also found physical activity was inversely associated with depression symptoms (e.g. Loprinzi 2011; Loprinzi et al. 2013; Bustamantea et al. 2013). They obtained minute by minute accelerometry data during the study, but their subsequent analysis only used the summary measures of sedentary, light, moderate, and vigorous activity levels over waking time. In fact, accelerometer data can also be used to examine patterns of physical activity throughout whole day and whole week, and can extract more detailed information than only summary statistics. To our knowledge, none of the previous studies have investigated the association between high frequency minute by minute physical activity data and depressive symptoms. Our study aims to explore different patterns between different depressive symptoms and can inform policy deliberation in the effort to improve the mental health and general health of targeted population.

2 Materials and Methods

2.1 Study Design and Participants

The Mitchelstown cohort was set up as a follow-up of the original Cork and Kerry cohort. Stratified random sampling by age and sex was utilised to recruit equal numbers of men and women between 50-69 years. Individuals with pre-existing cardiovascular disease or diabetes were not excluded. A total of 1018 people aged 50–69 attended for a study visit from 1473 who were invited to attend (response rate 69%). In 2011, recruitment was completed on a new cohort of 2047 men and women aged 50 to 69 years from patients attending a single large primary care centre, the Living Health Clinic in Mitchelstown (LHC), a town with a population of over 3,000 in county Cork. The LHC includes 8 general practitioners and the practice serves a catchment area of approximately 20,000 with a mix of urban and rural residents. Participants were randomly selected from all registered attending patients in the 50–69 years old age group. In total 2047 completed the questionnaire and physical examination components of the baseline assessment. Objective measurement of physical activity with the Geneactiv accelerometer was introduced in the later stages of the first wave of the study. Of the 765 participants who were asked to wear an accelerometer, 464 agreed (61% response rate), most of whom wore the accelerometer for the full 7 days, and finally we have 431 complete minute-by-minute accelerometer data. Taking consider of the length of wear time (larger than or equal to 10 h) in waking time (6:00 AM–12:00 PM) per day and background information, eventually 375 (87%) participants were included in this study.

2.2 Measurements

Assessment of Physical Activity. Wrist worn accelerometers measure the frequency and intensity of physical activity. Each participant was asked to wear an accelerometer, tri-axial Geneactive accelerometer for a period of 7 days. The accelerometers are waterproof and can be worn 24 h a day and they were set to record at 100 Hz, or 100 readings a second, for 7 days. This will ensure that 7 days of data is obtained from each participant. Data was collapsed into 1 min, raw 100 Hz tri-axial data was summarized as signal magnitude vector data (svm$_{gs}$, gravity adjusted) (svm$_{gs} = \sum \left| \sqrt{x^2 + y^2 + z^2} - 1 \right|$, x, y and z was the separate average value over 1 min 60 readings).

During data processing, it was important to identify waking time and non-wear time. We defined the waking time as 6:00 AM to 12:00 PM. Wear/non-wear time was determined using the van Hess et al. (2011) algorithm based on x-, y-, and z-axis 30 min standard deviations (<0.003 g) or 50 mg value range.

Assessment of Depression. Depression Scale (CES-D) (Radloff 1977): The CES-D is a widely used tool; it asks participants to report how frequently they had feelings or engaged in behaviors associated with depression in the previous week. Responses are made using a four-point scale spanning from 0 "Rarely or none of the time (<1 day)" to 3 "Most or all of the time (5–7 days)". A continuous total score is calculated based on

20 items with a possible range of 0 to 60; higher scores indicate more depressive symptoms. A CES-D score of 16 or higher has been demonstrated to correctly classify presence of depression in high percentages of older adults (Himmelfarb and Murrell 1983).

Other Measurements. Other covariates: age, gender, work status (work/retired or work at home) and BMI groups. BMI is a measure of weight adjusted for height and does not measure body composition directly. The WHO reported that, since 1980, the rates of obesity have increased threefold in Northern America, United Kingdom, Central and Eastern Europe, Pacific Island, Australia, and China (world health organization. Global strategy on diet, physical activity and health, world health organization. Geneva, Switzerland; 2004). The most common criteria's for defining weight status based on BMI are those recommended by the WHO. The WHO classification for BMI was utilized (underweight (<18.5 kg/m^2), normal weight (18.5–25 kg/m^2, reference category), overweight (25–30 kg/m^2) and obese (≥ 30 kg/m^2)) and BMI was entered as a categorical explanatory variable.

2.3   Statistical Analysis

Descriptive characteristics of the sample were presented as mean and standard deviation (SD) or median and quartiles for continuous variables, and frequency and percentage for categorical variables. The minute by minute activity levels was described using cubic splines smoothing method, which uses a set of polynomials of degree three and knots in the interval, then polynomial pieces fit together at knots, and its first and second derivatives are continuous at each knots, and hence on the whole interval.

Based on these analyses, the continuous relationship between log SVMgs and age was modeled using three multiple linear regression models with increased levels of adjustment for sex, body mass index (BMI), CESD score, employment status. Cubic spline smoothing was performed in R3.1.0. All the other analyses were carried out in SAS 9.3 (Statistical Analysis System Inc, 2002), $P \leq 0.05$ indicated statistically significance.

3   Results

3.1   Basic Characteristics of the Participants

Characteristic of the study sample by CESD depression groups is shown in Table 1. The mean age of the 375 subjects was 59.51 years (SD 5.48), with a range of 48.94–71.13 years, the mean body mass index of the 375 subjects was 28.88 (SD 4.56) kg/m^2, and with a range of 18.35 kg/m^2–48.44 kg/m^2. Of these, 202 (53.87%) were female, 173 (46.13%) were male, 180 (48%) work at home or retired and 195 (52%) were not retired. Table 1 was the description by depression groups.

Table 1. Descriptive characteristic of participants

Characteristics	None or minimal group	Mild	Moderate	Moderate to severe	p Value*
	(N = 207)	(N = 109)	(N = 36)	(N = 23)	
Age (years)	59.83 (5.39)	59.15 (5.57)	60.21 (5.45)	57.22 (5.53)	>0.05
Sex (male)	111 (96)	55 (54)	21 (15)	15 (8)	>0.05
BMI (kg/m^2)	28.66 (4.40)	28.96 (4.56)	29.75 (5.61)	29.04 (4.36)	>0.05
Work status (normal work)	89 (118)	49 (60)	26 (10)	16 (7)	<0.05

Note: *p value for group comparisons, analysis of variance for continuous measure, and chi-square test for proportions.

3.2 Within Day Physical Activity Profile

Physical activity profiles for one day using the original data averaged on every minute over 5 weekdays were shown in Figs. 1 and 2. Figure 1a is for participants in the different depression groups: none or minimal group, mild, moderate group, moderate to severe group; Fig. 1b is smoothed median activity for four depression groups: none or minimal (solid line), mild (dot line), moderate (dot-dashed line), moderate to severe (dashed line). After 11:00 pm and before around 7:00 am, participants in moderate and moderate to severe depression groups are much active than the other two groups, but during the other day time, moderate to severe group is less active than the others. Although daily activity tended to initiate between 7 and 8 am regardless of CESD groups. There were strong contrasts between depression groups regarding time-of day of peak per minute activity. Additionally, median activity intensity has almost two different peaks: "morning peak" and "afternoon peak" for all these four depression groups, the first peak occurs between 10 am and 12 pm and the second occurs between 4 pm and 6 pm. The cumulative activity intensity per day is shown in Fig. 2 by different depression groups. Daily activity gets progressively lower for moderate to severe group since between 7 am and 8 am, and the cumulative activity is the lowest among these four groups.

3.3 Bivariate Relationship Analysis of Confounders and Physical Activity

In general, from Fig. 3, time point "a" (about 1–2 am) to time point "b" (about 4 pm), male have much more than females. For 65 and under 65 years old people (midnight-5 pm = about 17 h), male have much more than females; except this period, female have much more than males (the difference is much smaller). For 65 and above, from about midnight—12 am = about 12 h, male have much more than females (but the difference is tiny); except this period, female have much more than males. Some interaction between age and gender; age getting older, the difference between female and male getting larger, from negative to positive. In general, from Fig. 4, CESD getting

(a)

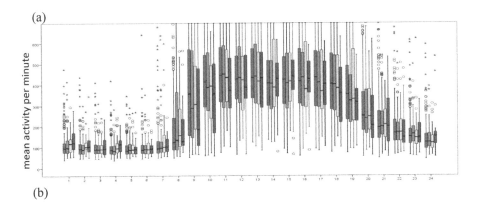

(b)

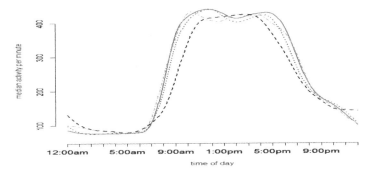

Fig. 1. Sample profiles for one day using the original data. (a) is by different depression groups (boxes from left to right: dep1-none or minimal group, dep2-mild, dep3-moderate, dep4-moderate to severe); (b) is smoothed median profiles for four depression groups: dep1-none or minimal (solid line), dep2-mild (dot line), dep3-moderate (dot-dashed line), dep4-moderate to severe (dashed line)

larger, participants tend to be less active. The maximum difference between non-depression and depression lies in 7–8 am. Getting older, the difference between non-depression and depression getting larger. For 65 and under 65 years old people (midnight-2.5 pm = about 2.5 h), depression people have much more than non-depression; except this period, non-depression have much more than depression. For 65 and above, non-depression people are much more active than depression. Some interaction between age and CESD score; age getting older, the difference between non-depression and depression getting larger.

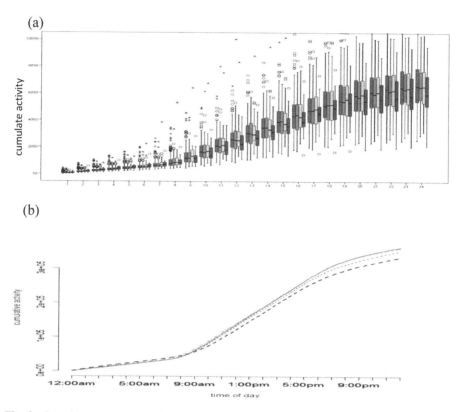

Fig. 2. Sample cumulative activity profiles per day by different depression groups. (a) boxes from left to right: none or minimal group, mild, moderate, moderate to severe); (b) is smoothed cumulative activity profiles for four depression groups: none or minimal (solid line), mild (dot line), moderate (dot-dashed line), moderate to severe (dashed line)

3.4 Regression Analysis

Time was divided into five different periods in one whole day (0–6, 6–12, 12–16, 16–20, 20–24). Median log svm_{gs} of each participant based on these five periods across five weekdays and weekends was obtained separately, five regression analysis was carried out then. Depression status was assessed using cutoff point of 17. The other covariates were also taken into considerations, such as age, BMI, sex and employment status (retired or not). The result showed that during 6 am–12 am, and 4 pm–12 am, CESD status had significantly negative effect on physical activity during weekdays. During the weekend, the significantly negative effect was found almost in all the daytime from 6 am–8 pm as shown in Fig. 5.

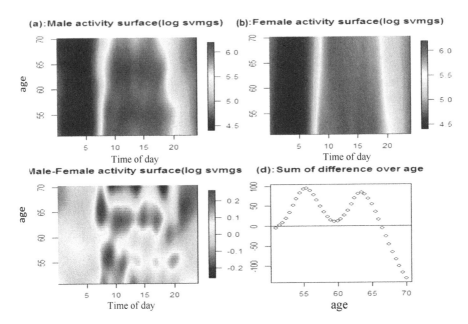

Fig. 3. Heat maps of estimated activity surfaces of males and females difference

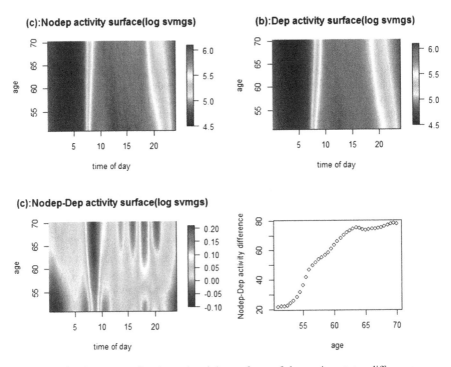

Fig. 4. Heat maps of estimated activity surfaces of depression status difference

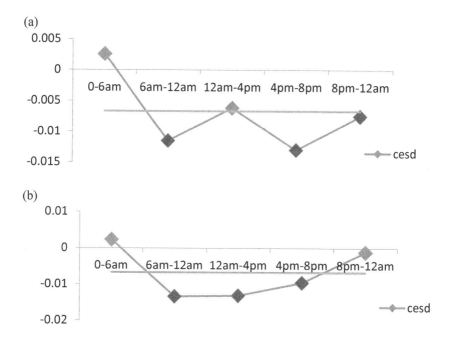

Fig. 5. Regression analysis for CESD and PA. (a) weekdays result, red color indicates the CESD status coefficient in this time points is significant comparted to the whole participants; (b) weekends result, the same explanation as weekdays (Color figure online)

4 Conclusion

Physical activity was affected by depression statuses, not only in daytime physical activity, but also in the early morning or late night activity. The activity profiles also varied depend on age, gender and weekday or weekend.

Acknowledgements. This project is funded by an Interdisciplinary Capacity Enhancement (ICE) Award provided by the Health Research Board, Ireland.

References

Babyak, M., et al.: Exercise treatment for major depression: maintenance of therapeutic benefit at 10 months. Psychosom. Med. **62**, 633–638 (2000)

Blumenthal, J.A., et al.: Cardiovascular and behavioural effects of aerobic exercise training in healthy older men and women. J. Gerontol. **44**, M147–M157 (1989)

Brown, D.R., et al.: Chronic psychological effects of exercise and exercise plus cognitive strategies. Med. Sci. Sport Exer. **27**, 765–775 (1995)

Brown, W.J., Ford, J.H., Burton, N.W., Marshall, A.L., Dobson, A.J.: Prospective study of physical activity in middle-aged women. Am. J. Prev. Med. **29**, 265–272 (2005)

Charlson, M.E., Pompei, P., Ales, K.L., MacKenzie, C.R.: A new method of classifying prognostic comorbidity in longitudinal studies: development and validation. J. Chronic Dis. **40**, 373–383 (1987)

DiLorenzo, T.M., Bargman, E.P., Stucky-Ropp, R., Brassington, G.S., Frensch, P.A., LaFontaine, T.: Long-term effects of aerobic exercise on psychological outcomes. Prev. Med. **28**, 75–85 (1999)

Bustamantea, E.E., Wilburb, J., Marqueza, D.X., Fogga, L., Staffilenob, B.A., Manning, A.: Physical activity characteristics and depressive symptoms in older Latino adults. Ment. Health Phys. Act. **6**(2), 69–77 (2013)

Emery, C.F., Blumenthal, J.A.: Effects of exercise training on psychological functioning in healthy type A men. Psychol. Health **2**, 367–379 (1988)

Foley, L.S., Prapavessis, H., Osuch, E.A., Pace, J.A.D., Murphy, B.A., Podolinsky, N.J.: An examination of potential mechanisms of exercise as a treatment for depression: a pilot study. Ment. Health Phys. Act. **7**(1), 69–73 (2008)

Hassmen, P., Koivula, N., Uutela, A.: Physical exercise and psychological well-being: a population study in Finland. Prev. Med. **30**, 17–25 (2000)

Himmelfarb, S., Murrell, S.A.: Reliability and validity of five mental health scales in older persons. J. Gerontol. **38**(3), 333–339 (1983)

Kalyani, R.R., Saudek, C.D., Brancati, F.L., Selvin, E.: Association of diabetes, comorbidities, and A1C with functional disability in older adults: results from the National Health and Nutrition Examination Survey (NHANES), 1999–2006. Diabetes Care **33**(5), 1055–1060 (2010)

Kessler, R.C., Ustun, T.B.: The WHO World Mental Health Surveys: Global Perspectives on the Epidemiology of Mental Disorders. Cambridge University Press, New York (2008)

King, A.C., Taylor, C.B., Haskell, W.L.: Effects of differing intensities and formats of 12 months of exercise training on psychological outcomes in older adults. Health Psychol. **12**, 292–300 (1993)

Klein, M.H., et al.: A comparative outcome study of group psychotherapy vs. exercise treatments for depression. Int. J. Ment. Health **13**, 148–177 (1985)

Moses, J., Steptoe, A., Mathews, A., Edwards, S.: The effects of exercise training on mental well-being in the normal population: a controlled trial. J. Psychosom. Res. **33**, 47–61 (1989)

Mota-Pereira, J., Silverio, J., Carvalho, S., Ribeiro, J.C., Fonte, D., Ramos, J.: Moderate exercise improves depression parameters in treatment-resistant patients with major depression disorder. J. Psychiatr. Res. **45**, 1005–1011 (2011)

Paffenbarger, R.S., Lee, I.M., Leung, R.: Physical activity and personal characteristics associated with depression and suicide in American college men. Acta Psychiatr. Scand. **337**(Suppl), 16–22 (1994)

Loprinzi, P.D.: Objectively measured light and moderate-to-vigorous physical activity is associated with lower depression levels among older US adults. Aging Ment. Health **17**(7), 801–805 (2011)

Loprinzi, P.D., Franz, C., Hagerc, K.: Accelerometer-assessed physical activity and depression among U.S. adults with diabetes. Ment. Health Phys. Act. **6**(2), 79–82 (2013)

Quan, H., et al.: Coding algorithms for defining comorbidities in ICD-9-CM and ICD-10 administrative data. Med. Care **43**, 1130–1139 (2005)

Radloff, L.S.: The CES-D Scale: a self-report depression scale for research in the general population. Appl. Psychol. Meas. **1**(3), 385–401 (1977)

Thirlaway, K., Benton, D.: Participation in physical activity and cardiovascular fitness have different effects on mental health and mood. J. Psychosom. Res. **36**, 657–665 (1992)

Wise, L.A., Adams-Cambell, L.L., Palmer, J.R., Rosenberg, L.: Leisuretime physical activity in relation to depressive symptoms in the black women's health study. Ann. Behav. Med. **32**, 384–392 (2006)

World Health Organization (WHO): Mental Health: A Call for Action by World Health Ministers. WHO Press, Geneva (2001)

World Health Organization (WHO): The Global Burden of Disease: 2004 Update. WHO Press, Geneva (2008)

World Health Organization (WHO): Media Center: Depression (2012). http://www.who.int/mediacentre/factsheets/fs369/en/index.html. Accessed 21 Feb 2013

Vallance, J.K., Winkler, E.A., Gardiner, P.A., Healy, G.N., Lynch, B.M., Owen, N.: Associations of objectively-assessed physical activity and sedentary time with depression: NHANES (2005–2006). Prev Med. **53**(4–5), 284–288 (2011)

Young, D.R., Sharp, D.S., Petrovitch, H., Curb, J.D.: Internal validity of the physical activity index over 26 years in middle-aged and older men. J. Am. Geriatr. Soc. **49**, 999–1006 (1995)

Detection of Depression from Brain Signals: A Review Study

Prabhjyot Kaur, Siuly Siuly$^{(\boxtimes)}$, and Yuan Miao

Centre for Applied Informatics, College of Engineering and Science,
Victoria University, Melbourne, VIC, Australia
prabhjyot.kaur@live.vu.edu.au,
{siuly.siuly, Yuan.Miao}@vu.edu.au

Abstract. Depression is a very common brain disorder now these days. It normally affects 10-15% of the population in the world. The untreated depression may lead to various undesirable consequences such as suicide, poor physical health, self-harm, etc. There is no age group left behind from this disorder. Depression affects negatively on an individual's personal, professional and social life. Detection of depression from brain signals (Such as Electroencephalogram (EEG)) is a challenging task for both research and neurologist due to the non-stationary and chaotic nature of EEG signals. The depression detection at an early stage is very important because it can help patients to obtain the best treatment on time and we can prevent them from harmful consequences. Aim of this study is to provide the current scenery of detection of depression from EEG signals. The EEG signals use as a tool to read the brain activity of an individual. The results of EEG test help us to perform the different techniques to detect the depression. In addition, this paper provides the general idea of different stages of depression detection such as the data collection, pre-processing, feature extraction- selection and classification, it also reports the existing techniques in this area. End of this work, finally we can find the limitations of existing work and the directions for future work.

Keywords: Electroencephalogram · K-nearest neighbors
Support Vector Machine · Probabilistic Neural Network
Naive Bayes Classifier

1 Introduction

Depression is an unbearable state for any human being that affects their abilities to work, think and in their behavior. It is causing a lot of physical and mental health problems which affects the family and social life of an individual in a negative way. Sadly, the depression becomes a common mental disorder now these days. Depression is the most important reason for mental disorder worldwide. In Australia, every year 1 person out of 5 people experiences a mental illness [1]. In America, nearly 6.7% population are affected by mental illness every year [2]. According to the Australian Bureau of Statistics, over 40% of the individual (male and female) will experience mental illness during their life [3]. Suicide is the worst result of depression. According to the reports if depressive patients will not get treated the chances of suicide is placed

© Springer Nature Switzerland AG 2018
S. Siuly et al. (Eds.): HIS 2018, LNCS 11148, pp. 48–57, 2018.
https://doi.org/10.1007/978-3-030-01078-2_5

at 20% [4]. The Australian cost of depression is $14.9 billion in 2012 [5]. Depression can be treated if detected, but unfortunately, only 20% of people with depressive illness got treated because of the unawareness of depression [6]. Beyond Blue and Black Dog institutes educating peoples for depression symptoms, to seek the treatment and look out for others to depression [1, 5]. We believe an automatic tool for depression detection improves health care for patients and the working environment for practitioners. A tool cannot replace the doctor, psychologist or psychiatrist but it can help them to support their decisions.

Electroencephalography (EEG) is a tool to measure the electrical activity of the human brain [7, 24, 25]. It is a popular test that provides evidence of how the brain functions in a period. The EEG is widely used by doctors and researchers to study brain functions, which helps them to detect neural disorders [7]. EEG signal is also called brain signal that contain huge volumes of data with dynamic characteristics (e.g. aperiodic, non-stationary and nonlinear) [26, 27, 29, 32]. So far, the EEG data are visually analysed by experts to identify and understand depression within the brain and how they propagate [28]. Manual approach to analysing huge data is an inefficient and inaccurate procedure (e.g. time and resource-consuming, and human error contributes to reduced decision-making reliability) [30, 31, 33].

Most of the researches use a typical approach for detecting and classifying depression activities from EEG that includes some general steps shown in Fig. 1. Figure 1 illustrates a universal block diagram of the EEG signal classification used in almost all papers. The first step of any research is to collect the data from different sources such as collect data from an individual by using EEG machine or using pre-collected data from any hospital or from any open source database. As we discuss before that EEG data have some unwanted information, so the second step is to clean the data from unnecessary information and used that as an input for the third step which is features extraction and selection. In features extraction and selection step normally, the representative features are extracted and selected. It can be based on two types frequency such as alpha, delta, beta etc. and another one is time series, such a variance, max power, and sum power etc. the feature extraction is depending upon the research requirements. The selected features then classified on different classifiers such as k-nearest neighbors (KNN) [34, 35], Support Vector Machine (SVM) [34, 36], Probabilistic Neural Network (PNN) and Naive Bayes Classifier (NBC) [37] etc. Classification method then helps in the decision-making process to declare that the person is depressed or not.

The rest of the paper divided into seven section. The second section is EEG data collection where we discuss the data collection techniques and compare them a little bit. Whereas in section three we pre-processed the collected data and the importance of pre-processing of the data and provide some literature in pre-processing. The sections four and five are discussed the feature extraction, selection and classification of EEG signals and some existing methods are discussed. Section six is discussion and seven concludes the paper.

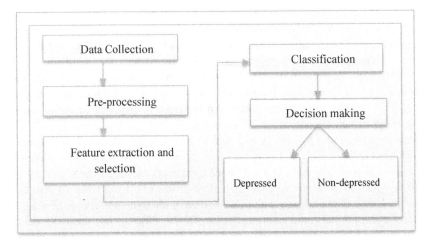

Fig. 1. General framework from EEG signals

2 EEG Data Collection

The depression EEG data has been collected by placing the electrode on the scalp or by Three-electrode pervasive device. The data is collected in a dark and quiet room with a laydown position of an individual. The two different methods of collecting EEG data are shown in Figs. 2 and 3. Whereas the Three electrode Placement device is easy to use and provide the same results with less hassle [8].

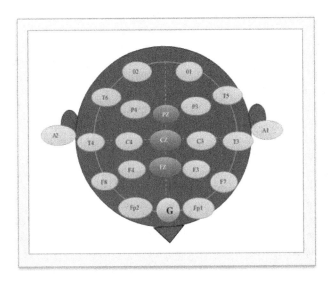

Fig. 2. International 10–20 system electrode placement

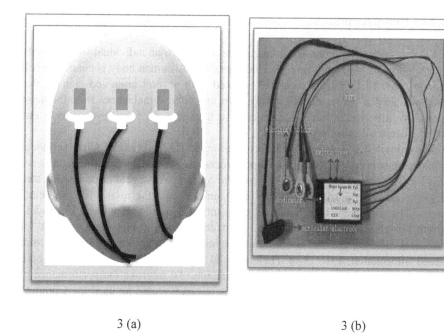

3 (a)   3 (b)

Fig. 3. Three-electrode pervasive EEG collection device

Figure 2 shows the International 10–20 system where electrodes placed on an individual's scalp for collecting the data. The collector must adjust the electrodes during the coaction process to obtain the better results [8]. This method is not only very hard and time-consuming, but it is tried for the patient as well. This method only used in the advanced hospitals or institutes.

In Fig. 3(a) we show the position of electrodes placed in a human's forehead whereas in Fig. 3(b) we show the actual image of three- electrodes pervasive device. This device has been developed by the UAIS lab. In this device, the approximate length of the cable is 25 cm and it can also use batteries, which makes this device very convenient for users. For the data transmission, the device uses the Bluetooth facility [9].

The three-electrode pervasive EEG collection method is more effective and easier for use and the patient as comparative to the traditional 10–20 electrode system. The 3-electrode pervasive methods are quicker than the other as in other methods the collector must adjust the electors during the collection process there are so many electrodes which takes more time comparing the 3 electrodes.

3 EEG Pre-processing

The EEG data collection process is a long process in which an individual sit in a comfy chair or lay down on a bed during the whole process. A human body is cannot be still for a long time. EEG data is naturally polluted with several uninvited signals, that affects the quality of the results negatively. This uninvited signal comes from the noise composed by different physical movements such as muscle, head, eye or teeth etc. During the data collection process [10]

These uninvited signals called artifacts and noise. The process of removing these uninvited signals is called de-noising or pre-processing. In this process, the signals are cleaned form uninvited signals and prepare them for the next stage. Pre-processing step is very important because noise or artifacts can decrease the quality of the actual outcomes. This step helps to extract maximum information of data without destroying important signals. There are several ways to denoise the data before using it for research and different authors use different techniques to denoise their signals from unwanted information. Liao et al. [11] believed that raw EEG signals have a poor resolution because of the volume conduction effects. To improve the performance of the signals, spatial filtering is necessary. In his research paper, he used the Common Spatial Pattern (CSP) technique and prove that CSP is better than other spatial filters such as bipolar and common average reference filters [11]. Matiko et al. [12] present a method of removing the noise in EEG signals by using Morphological Component analysis (MCA) method. MCA fast computation of signal coefficients and it requires less memory [12]. Rachman et al. [13] used the Independent Component Analysis (ICA) to remove the inaccurate information caused by some movements such as eye blinking, heart signals and a wink etc. this method works as a blind source separation by breaks data into a form which is called independent component [13]. The components corresponding to the BCG are identified by visual inspection or by a correlation analysis with the EEG signal [14].

K. Lakshmi et al. [15] research to compare four methods to de-noise the EEG data form artifacts. In their research, they perform the denoise process on EEG using principal component analysis (PCA), ICA, Butterworth filter and FIR filter algorithms. In their research, they find that the ICA is the most appropriate method with the least errors [15].

Some authors use principal component analysis (PCA) and template-based algorithms. The PCA-based methods work with BCG artefact. It is identifying its principal components, fitting them to the EEG signal, and then take away the fitted model of the artefacts. ICA-based methods discrete the signal into independent source components [14].

This step assures the researcher to achieve the more accurate outcome as compared to use raw data for further steps. Different authors used different methods to denoised their data but according to Lakshmi et al. ICA is the most accurate result provider method. The pre-processed signals will use as an input for the next step.

4 Feature Extraction and Selection

Feature extraction is a process of transformation of the large volume of input data into important features sets where the probabilities of loose the important information are too low. It makes the analysis process fast and easy. Feature extraction means to determine a systematic path from the regular pre-processed data signals. A feature could be some characteristic measurements such as based in time or frequency or structural element extracted from a pattern section. The two major units of conventional feature extraction modules are statistical characteristic and syntactic descriptions. Feature extraction part is processed to select the most important features or information from the EEG signals for classification part [16].

The feature extraction part performs a major importance to achieve the accuracy in the research. The classification step will be performed on the data extracted and selected in this step and analysis the results based on extracted features. This is the major area to concentrate for any investigator to choose what feature would be extracted and select in regarding achieve the desired outcome.

Wu et al. [17] extract the sensorimotor area feature from EEG data using Spatial Filtering methods [17]. The study by Li et al. [18] filtered EEG signals with Hanning Filter to extract the frequency bands. The extracted frequency band are delta frequency from 0.5 Hz to 4 Hz, theta 4 Hz to 8 Hz, alpha range from 8 Hz to 13 Hz and beta from 13 Hz to 30 Hz. used nonlinear method for feature extraction. The author extract twelve linear features in time series, such a variance, max power, and sum power etc. for each electrode of the 128 channels [18]. Faust et al. [19] introduced a processing structure for depression detection. In this research, the author divides the feature extraction process into two steps. First, WPD was used to extract an appropriate sub-band from the EEG signal. In the second step, the resulting sub-band signals were used as input for non-linear feature extraction algorithms. The different non- linear measure employing entropy methods to extract the features of nonlinear methods are approximate entropy (ApEn), sample entropy (SampEn), renyi entropy (REN) and bispectral phase entropy (Ph). Entropy is a theoretical framework, which measures of uncertainty, or regularity of a signal. To analyse the collected data of 30 individuals, the authors used the classical feature extraction method. The nonlinear feature extraction was applied with the help of different entropies methods [19]. Achara et al. [20] proposed a system based on nonlinear features for depression diagnosis in EEG signals. This paper used nonlinear methods such as fractal dimension, largest Lyapunov exponent, sample entropy, detrended fluctuation analysis, Hurst's exponent, higher order spectra, and recurrence quantification for analysis [20]. H M [21] provide a noble approach for depression level prediction in this research. To predict the level of depression they used the Welch method to extract the features of EEG data. This method extracts the features based on frequency bands such as alpha, theta and delta from pre-processed data [21]. A study by Li et al. [18] adopt Correlation-based Feature Selection (CFS) method and used BestFirst method for search. The CFS selects a subset of features that are highly correlated with the class while having low intercorrelation, which helps to recognise the location of the electrode which has the strong correlation with depression [18].

5 Classification

The classification is a process to differentiate the unknown test set into their appropriate class. The extracted features become the input for this step. This step majors the performance of classifiers and provides the results. The most commonly used classifiers for EEG signals are KNN, NBC, PNN and SVM. A research by Li et al. [17] employed five representative classifiers from different types including methods based on distance such as KNN, functional based method Logistic Regression and SVM has been used [18]. On the other side Faust et al. [19] used 7 different classification algorithms such as Gaussian Mixture Model (GMM), Discrete Transformation (DT), KNN, NBC, PNN and SVM for classification process. This paper obtained a classification accuracy of 99.5%, sensitivity 99.2% and specificity of 99.7% using PNN classifier [19]. Bachmann et al. [22] proposed an idea for depression detection from EEG, which focused on linear Spectral Asymmetry Index (SASI) and non-linear Detrended Fluctuation Analysis (DFA) methods. The results show that the linear combination of SASI and DFA achieved higher classification accuracy with 91.2%, where the SASI got 76.5% and DFA got 70.6% respectively [22]. Achara et al. [20] ranked the nonlinear extracted features and fed to the SVM classifier for results [20]. H M [21] use the Adaptive Neuro-fuzzy Inference system (ANFIS) and Neural Network Pattern Recognition Tool (nprtool) for the classification of the parameters extracted and selected from previous steps [21].

S. Puthankattil et al. [23] applied feedforward neural network (FFNN) and PNN methods two networks to evaluate the performance is EEG signals of normal and depressive patients in their study. Their study shows that the classification accuracy of FFNN is much superior to PNN in depression signals [23].

6 Discussion

In the order to examine the different techniques of data collection we find that the three electrodes placement method is easy for both parties (the examiner and the patient) as compared to the traditional international 10–20 one. In the other sections of the paper shows that most of the papers use the traditional machine learning methods for feature extraction, selection and classification such as KNN, SVM, NBC etc. these traditional methods can't process EEG signals at higher and deeper level [20]. This limitation can be solved by using deep learning methods, it may be possible to get more accurate results by adopting the deep learning approaches over traditional machine learning methods.

7 Conclusions

This paper presents the exciting research in this area to find the directions for further research. In this article, a review of EEG-based diagnosis of depression is presented with a feature extraction, selection and classification methods. The literature reveals that every method has their own advantages and disadvantages which, makes them appropriate for some specific kind of researches. After reviewing the literature, the existing methods has the various limitations, so we decide to use the deep learning methods over the traditional machine learning methods.

Our project will offer considerable importance in the medical field and provide help in treatment approaches of depression. The manual study of the EEG reports is a time consuming and expensive task, this project will save the time and cost of the EEG manual study. It is hoped that the output of this research will be a great milestone for the medical field. These obtained findings may have the generalizability to provide an effective approach for depression diagnosis and to help depressed patients take precautions early and this will turn enhance the overall welfare of patients.

References

1. Black Dog Institute: Facts and figures about mental health and mood disorders (2012). http://www.blackdoginstitute.org.au/docs/Factsandfiguresaboutmentalhealthandmooddisorders.pdf
2. National Institute of Mental Health (USA): The numbers count: Mental disorders in America (2013). http://www.nimh.nih.gov/health/publications/the-numbers-count-mental-disorders-in-america/index.shtml
3. The Australian Bureau of Statistics: Mental health (2009). http://www.ausstats.abs.gov.au/ausstats/subscriber.nsf/LookupAttach/4102.0Publication25.03.094/$File/41020Mentalhealth.pdf
4. Gotlib, I., Hammen, C.: Handbook of Depression. Guilford Press, New York (2002)
5. Beyond Blue: The facts: depression and anxiety (2012). http://www.beyondblue.org.au/the-facts
6. Murray, B., Fortinberry, A.: Depression facts and stats (2005). http://www.upliftprogram.com/depressionstats.html
7. Siuly, S., Li, Y., Zhang, Y.: EEG Signal Analysis and Classification: Techniques and Applications. Health Information Science. Springer, Heidelberg (2016). https://doi.org/10.1007/978-3-319-47653-7. ISBN 978-3-319-47653-7
8. Shen, J., Zhao, S., Yao, Y., Wang, Y., Feng, L.: A novel depression detection method based on pervasive EEG and EEG splitting criterion. In: IEEE International Conference on Bioinformatics and Biomedicine (BIBM), pp. 1879–1886 (2017)
9. Cai, H., Sha, X., Han, X., Wei, S., Hu, B.: Pervasive EEG diagnosis of depression using deep belief network with three-electrodes eeg collector. In: IEEE International Conference on Bioinformatics and Biomedicine (BIBM), pp. 1239–1246 (2016)
10. da Cruz, J., Chicherov, V., Herzog, M., Figueiredo, P.: An automatic pre-processing pipeline for EEG analysis (APP) based on robust statistics. Clin. Neurophysiol. **129**(7), 1427–1437 (2018)
11. Liao, S., Wu, C., Huang, H., Cheng, W., Liu, Y.: Major depression detection from EEG signals using Kernel Eigen-Filter-Bank common spatial patterns. Sensors **17**(6), 1385 (2017)
12. Matiko, J., Beeby, S., Tudor, J.: Real time eye blink noise removal from EEG signals using morphological component analysis. In: 35th Annual International Conference of the IEEE EMBS Osaka, Japan, pp. 13–16 (2013)
13. Rachman, N., Tjandrasa, H., Fatichah, C.: Alcoholism classification based on EEG data using Independent Component Analysis (ICA), wavelet de-noising and Probabilistic Neural Network (PNN). In: International Seminar on Intelligent Technology and Its Application (2016)

14. Schulz, M., et al.: On utilizing uncertainty information in template-based EEG-fMRI ballistocardiogram artifact removal. Psychophysiology 52(6), 857–863 (2015)
15. Lakshmi, K., Surling, S., Sheeba, O.: A novel approach for the removal of artifacts in EEG signals (2017)
16. Al-Fahoum, A., Al-Fraihat, A.: Methods of EEG signal features extraction using linear analysis in frequency and time-frequency domains. ISRN Neurosci. 1–7 (2014)
17. Liu, Y.-T., et al.: Fuzzy integral with particle swarm optimization for a motor-imagery-based brain computer interface. IEEE Trans. Fuzzy Syst. 25, 21–28 (2016)
18. Li, X., Hu, B., Shen, J., Xu, T., Retcliffe, M.: Mild depression detection of college students: an EEG-based solution with free viewing tasks. J. Med. Syst. 39(12), 187 (2015)
19. Faust, O., Ang, P., Puthankattil, S., Joseph, P.: Depression diagnosis support system based on EEG signal entropies. J. Mech. Med. Biol. 14(03), 1450035 (2014)
20. Acharya, U., et al.: A novel depression diagnosis index using nonlinear features in EEG signals. Eur. Neurol. 74(1–2), 79–83 (2015)
21. Mallikarjun, H.M., Suresh, D.: Depression level prediction using EEG signal processing. In: International Conference on Contemporary Computing and Informatics, IC (2014)
22. Bachmann, M., Lass, J., Hinrikus, H.: Single channel EEG analysis for detection of depression. Biomed. Signal Process. Control 31, 391–397 (2017)
23. Puthankattil, S., Joseph, P.: Half-wave segment feature extraction of EEG signals of patients with depression and performance evaluation of neural network classifiers. J. Mech. Med. Biol. 17(01), 1750006 (2017)
24. Kabir, E., Siuly, S., Cao, J., Wang, H.: A computer aided analysis scheme for detecting epileptic seizure from EEG data. Int. J. Comput. Intell. Syst. 11(1), 663–671 (2018)
25. Siuly, S., Wang, H., Zhang, Y.: Detection of motor imagery EEG signals employing Naïve Bayes based learning process. Measurement 86, 148–158 (2016)
26. Supriya, S., Siuly, S., Wang, H., Zhang, Y.: An efficient framework for the analysis of big brain signals data. In: ADC 2018: Databases Theory and Applications, pp. 199–207 (2018)
27. Siuly, S., Kabir, E., Wang, H., Zhang, Y.: Exploring sampling in the detection of multi category EEG signals. In: Computational and Mathematical Methods in Medicine, pp. 1–12 (2015)
28. Siuly, S., Zhang, Y.: Medical big data: neurological diseases diagnosis through medical data analysis. Data Sci. Eng. 1(2), 54–64 (2016)
29. Siuly, S., Zarei, R., Wang, H., Zhang, Y.: A new data mining scheme for analysis of big brain signal data. In: ADC 2017: Databases Theory and Applications, pp. 151–164 (2017)
30. Supriya, S., Siuly, S., Cao, J., Zhang, Y.: Weighted visibility graph with complex network features in the detection of epilepsy. IEEE Access. 4, 6554–6566 (2016)
31. Supriya, S., Siuly, S., Wang, H., Zhuo G., Zhang, Y.: Analyzing EEG signal data for detection of epileptic seizure: introducing weight on visibility graph with complex network feature. In: ADC 2016: Databases Theory and Applications, pp. 56–66 (2016)
32. Hassan, A.R., Siuly, S., Zhang, Y.: Epileptic seizure detection in EEG signals using tunable-Q factor wavelet transform and Bootstrap aggregating. Comput. Methods Programs Biomed. 137, 247–259 (2016)
33. Alçïn, Ö.F., Siuly, S., Bajaj, V., Guo, Y., Şengur, A., Zhang, Y.: Multi-category EEG signal classification developing time-frequency texture features based fisher vector encoding method. Neurocomputing 218, 51–258 (2016)
34. Siuly, S., Yin, X., Hadjiloucas, S., Zhang, Y.: Classification of THz pulse signals using two-dimensional cross-correlation feature extraction and non-linear classifiers. Comput. Methods Programs Biomed. 127, 64–82 (2016)
35. Kabir, E., Siuly, S., Zhang, Y.: Epileptic seizure detection from EEG signals using logistic model trees. Brain Inform. 3(2), 93–100 (2016)

36. Al Ghayab, H.R., Li, Y., Siuly, S., Abdulla, S.: Epileptic EEG signal classification using optimum allocation based power spectral density estimation. IET Signal Proc. **12**(6), 738–747 (2018)
37. Siuly, S., Li, Y.: Discriminating the brain activities for brain–computer interface applications through the optimal allocation-based approach. Neural Comput. Appl. **26**(4), 799–811 (2014)

Artificial Intelligence for Computer-aided Diagnosis

Extreme Learning Machine Based Diagnosis Models for Erythemato-Squamous Diseases

Juanying Xie[1]([⊠]) [ORCID], Xinyuan Ji[1], and Mingzhao Wang[2]

[1] School of Computer Science, Shaanxi Normal University,
Xi'an 710119, People's Republic of China
xiejuany@snnu.edu.cn
[2] College of Life Science, Shaanxi Normal University,
Xi'an 710119, People's Republic of China

Abstract. Extreme learning machine based features selection algorithms are proposed in this paper for diagnosing erythemato-squamous diseases. The algorithms adopt the traditional ELM (extreme learning machine), EM-ELM (the error minimum extreme learning machine) and K-ELM (kernel extreme learning machine), respectively, to evaluate the power of the detected feature subset. The improved F-score and SFS (sequential forward search) strategy are combined to detect feature subsets. To detect a much more accurate diagnosis model for erythemato-squamous diseases, an ensemble diagnosis model is constructed by combining three models (classifiers) built on three feature subsets detected by proposed feature selection algorithms respectively. 5-fold cross validation experiments are conducted to test the performance of each feature selection algorithm, and the ensemble model. Experimental results demonstrate that the ensemble model has got the best accuracy. Its highest and average classification accuracy in 5-fold cross validation experiments are 100% and 98.31%, respectively.

Keywords: Extreme learning machine
Error minimum extreme learning machine
Kernel extreme learning machine · Feature selection
Improved F-score · Erythemato-squamous disease

1 Introduction

It is a very challengeable thing for medical doctors to make proper diagnosis for patients with erythemato-squamous diseases. The first reason of this is that there are all six groups in erythemato-squamous diseases, including

Supported by NSFC under Grant No. 61673251 & by Fundamental Research Funds for Central Universities under Grant No. GK201701006 & by the Innovation Funds of Graduate Programs at Shaanxi Normal University under Grant No. 2015CXS028 and 2016CSY009.

S. Siuly et al. (Eds.): HIS 2018, LNCS 11148, pp. 61–74, 2018.
https://doi.org/10.1007/978-3-030-01078-2_6

psoriasis (PS), seborrheic dermatitis (SD), lichen planus (LP), pityriasis rosea (PR), chronic dermatitis (CD) and pityriasis rubra pilaris (PRP), and the six groups of erythemato-squamous diseases share the clinical features of erythema and scaling with very little differences. Second, there are many common histopathological features and one disease may show features of another disease at the beginning stage and may have its own characteristic features at the following stages.

However, in recent decade, artificial intelligence (AI) has achieved great developments [15], and has been widely applied in many fields [16], especially in biomedical data analysis [7,27]. There have been many AI experts devoting themselves to the diagnosis study of erythemato-squamous diseases, such that many different machine learning approaches have been introduced to diagnose erythema-squamous diseases [13,17,21,22]. In order to help medical doctors to make proper diagnosis for patients of erythema-squamous diseases, there have been several feature selection algorithms have been proposed to detect the primary features of erythema-squamous diseases [10,14,23,26,28,29]. The latest research [10] in this field is that mRMR (minimum Redundancy Maximum Relevance) and ELM (Extreme Learning Machine) have been introduced to differential diagnosis of erythemato-squamous diseases, where mRMR [3] is adopted to implement feature selection process and ELM is used as a classifier. The method has got the highest and average classification accuracy of 98.89% and 98.55%, respectively, with 10-fold cross validation experiments. Although ELM is a very fast and accurate learning machine, mRMR is a time-consuming feature selection algorithm. Therefore we propose to use the improved F-score [28], a very fast method, and SFS (sequential forward search), an efficient strategy [24], together to implement feature selection procedure, so as to detect primary features of erythemato-squamous diseases in this paper. In addition, we propose to use tradition ELM [6], EM-ELM [4] and K-ELM [5] as classifiers, respectively, to guide the feature selection procedure, so as to get the powerful feature subset fast. Finally, we propose to combine the aforementioned ELM, EM-ELM and K-ELM based feature selection algorithms together to construct an ensemble model for diagnosing erythemato-squamous diseases by combining the three proposed models (classifiers). The performance of the proposed feature selection algorithms and the ensemble diagnosing model have been tested in 5-fold cross validation experiments on dermatology database.

This article is organized as follows. Section 2 introduces the main ideas of proposed feature selection algorithms and the ensemble model. Section 3 displays the experimental results and the analyses. Conclusions come in Sect. 4.

2   Proposed Algorithms

Let $\mathbf{X} = \{(\mathbf{x}_k, y_k) \mid \mathbf{x}_k \in \mathbf{R}^n, \ y_k \in \{1, \cdots, l\}, k = 1, \cdots, m\}$ be the dataset, where, n is the number of features, m is the number of samples, and l is the number of classes. We use the improved F-score proposed in [6] to evaluate the contribution of each feature to diagnosing erythema-squamous diseases, and SFS strategy to find feature subset, and traditional ELM [6] or EM-ELM [4]or K-ELM [5] as a classifier to value the power of the feature subset in diagnosing erythema-squamous diseases. 5-fold cross validation experiments have been conducted for each feature subset selection algorithm, and 10-fold cross validation experiments have been adopted for each fold to detect the optimal feature subset, on which to build the diagnosis model with high accuracy for erythema-squamous diseases. The main ideas of the three algorithms are described in Fig. 1. After that we construct an ensemble diagnosis model for erythema-squamous diseases by combing the three feature selection algorithms. Fig. 2 describes the idea of the ensemble model.

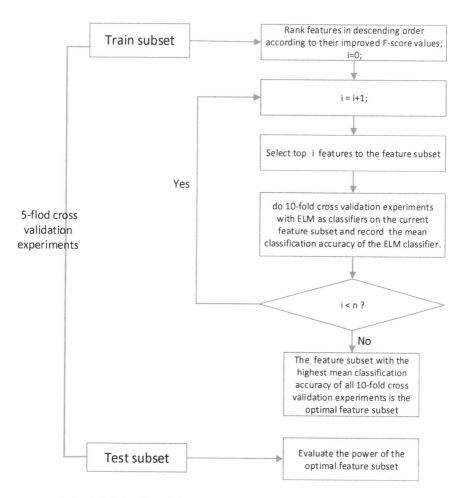

Fig. 1. Main idea of the proposed feature selection algorithms.

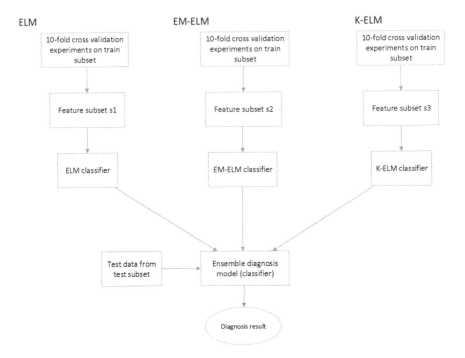

Fig. 2. Ensemble diagnosis model for erythemato-squamous diseases.

3   Experiments and Analyses

This section will introduce the dataset first, then the experimental results and analyses are followed.

3.1   Dataset

The dataset is from UCI Machine Learning Repository [2]. It has 366 samples while 8 samples are with missing values. We delete these 8 samples, and use the remaining 358 samples in our experiments. Each sample has 34 attributes. The 34th attribute is the patients' actual age. The 11th attribute is the patient's family history whose values take 1 or 0, respectively meaning that the diseases were observed in the patient family or not. The remaining 32 attributes are the clinical or histopathological attributes whose values are 0, 1, 2 or 3 respectively representing a degree in the range from 0 to 3, with 0 indicating the feature was not present, 3 the largest amount possible, and 1, 2 indicating the relative intermediate values. Column 35 of the dataset represents class labels with a total of six values, indicating the six types of erythemato-squamous diseases.

3.2   Experimental Results

For each feature selection algorithm, 5-fold cross validation experiments have been conducted. To find the optimal feature subset for each fold, 10-fold cross validation experiments have been done on train subset. The ensemble diagnosis model has been constructed by combing three classifiers based on ELM, EM-ELM and K-ELM, respectively. The result of the ensemble diagnosis model is obtained by majority voting strategy. The sigmoid activation function is adopted in ELM and EM-ELM based feature selection algorithms while the RBF (Radial Basis Function) is adopted by K-ELM as the activation function. Here we will describe the experimental results of each feature selection algorithm in detail, then the results of the ensemble model. Black fonts mean the best results in experiments.

ELM Based Feature Selection Algorithm. The performance of traditional ELM is variant with the number of its hidden nodes. Therefore we did 5-fold cross validation experiments without feature selection to study the relationship between the accuracy of ELM and its hidden nodes by varying the number of hidden nodes, so as to get the rough interval of nodes on which the ELM can obtain its high classification accuracy. After that we did ELM based feature selection algorithm, and compare the classification accuracy of ELM classifier with and without feature selection procedure. Figure 3 plots the curve of accuracy of ELM with its hidden nodes.

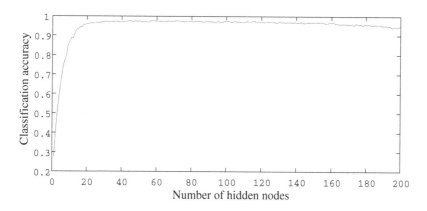

Fig. 3. The curve of classification accuracy with the hidden nodes in ELM.

The results in Fig. 3 disclose that the accuracy of ELM increases rapidly before its hidden nodes go up to 20, after that its accuracy enter into a roughly stable level. The highest accuracy comes when the number of hidden nodes are in the interval from 30 to 80. This fact discloses that the accuracy of ELM will not always go up with its hidden nodes, too many hidden nodes may lead to over-fitting. It is enough for ELM to have 55 hidden nodes.

Table 1 displays the results of ELM based feature selection algorithm. For each specific number of hidden nodes, we did 10-fold cross validation experiments on train subset to find the optimal feature subset, then built the classifier on the train subset, and recorded the test accuracy. The mean accuracy with standard deviation, mean numbers of features in feature subset, and the mean training time of 5-fold cross validation experiments are recorded in Table 1. Table 2 compare the results of ELM based feature selection algorithm with 75 hidden nodes and of ELM with 55 hidden nodes on original dataset without feature selection. Table 3 lists the feature subsets of 5-fold cross validation experiments of ELM based feature selection algorithm.

Table 1. Results of ELM based feature selection algorithm.

#hidden nodes	#selected features	accuracy/%	training time/s
5	11.4	77.3749 ± 5.2943	2.3781
15	23.8	94.6888 ± 0.6525	3.0688
25	25.6	96.9348 ± 2.4825	3.4781
35	25.6	96.4101 ± 2.7749	3.2094
45	26.2	96.6266 ± 1.6446	3.3625
55	24.8	97.4758 ± 1.5545	3.7375
65	25.6	97.2055 ± 0.9842	4.0594
75	**25.0**	**97.7615 ± 0.7758**	**5.4938**
85	26.2	97.1821 ± 1.7738	5.8031
95	24.4	97.1976 ± 1.0261	6.0906
105	26.6	96.9202 ± 1.8295	6.5875
125	26.0	96.9043 ± 1.2326	7.1656
150	29.0	96.6654 ± 1.5509	8.8094

It can be seen from the results in Table 1 that the ELM based feature selection algorithm can find the best feature subset with 25 features within 5.5 seconds in mean, when there are 75 hidden nodes in the network. The classifier on the feature subset has got the highest classification accuracy about 97.76% averagely.

Table 2 tells us that ELM based feature selection algorithm can get better classification accuracy with fewer features compared to that without feature selection process embedded. The mean accuracy is 97.7615%.

From the results in Table 3, we can see that features 1, 13, 17, 18 and 32 were not selected into any feature subset in 5-fold cross validation experiments, which means that these features are not significant to distinguish any specific erythemato-squamous disease.

Table 2. Comparison between ELM based feature selection and ELM.

| | ELM + improved F-score | | | ELM | |
folds	#features	Accuracy/%	Training time/s	#features	Accuracy/%
fold1	24	**98.6486**	5.5469	34	95.9054
fold2	22	**97.2222**	5.2969	34	95.3611
fold3	23	97.2222	5.4531	34	**98.0278**
fold4	28	**97.1429**	5.8906	34	96.6000
fold5	28	**98.5714**	5.2813	34	98.3000
mean	25	**97.7615**	5.4938	34	96.8389

Table 3. Feature subset by ELM based feature selection algorithm.

folds	Feature subset
fold1	5,6,7,8,9,10,12,14,15,16,20,21,22,23,24,25,26,27,28,29,30,31,33,34
fold2	5,6,7,8,9,10,12,14,15,16,20,21,22,24,25,26,27,28,29,30,31,33
fold3	5,6,7,8,9,10,12,14,15,16,20,21,22,24,25,26,27,28,29,30,31,33,34
fold4	2,3,4,5,6,7,8,9,10,12,14,15,16,19,20,21,22,23,24,25,26,27,28,29,30,31,33,34
fold5	2,3,4,5,6,7,8,9,10,11,12,14,15,16,20,21,22,23,24,25,26,27,28,29,30,31,33,34

EM-ELM Based Feature Selection Algorithm. It is well known that the number of hidden nodes affect the performance of ELM classifier. To get the best classification accuracy, we did experiments to find the best number of hidden nodes for ELM based feature selection algorithm, though it is a time-consuming process. Therefore we propose to use EM-ELM instead of ELM in feature selection process, so as to the hidden nodes will be determined automatically given the threshold of accuracy.

We first did 5-fold cross validation experiments on original dataset without feature selection when the threshold of EM-ELM was varied from 0.5 to 1. Table 4 displays the results including the threshold, average accuracy with standard deviation, and the mean number of hidden nodes. After that we studied the influence of threshold on EM-ELM based feature selection algorithm, and the results of 5-fold cross validation experiments were shown in Table 5, where the optimal feature subset for each fold was detected by 10-fold cross validation experiments on train subset given the specific threshold. Table 6 gives the results of EM-ELM based feature selection algorithms compared to that of EM-ELM without feature selection. Table 7 displays the feature subsets of 5-fold cross validation experiments on the dataset.

It can be seen from Table 4 that the performance of EM-ELM goes up with its threshold, and the number of hidden nodes also increases. However, when the threshold is 0.99, the EM-ELM has got its best performance with the relative number of hidden nodes.

Table 4. Performance of EM-ELM under specific threshold.

Threshold	Accuracy	Mean hidden nodes
0.5	65.2752 ± 0.0092	5.10
0.6	69.3221 ± 0.0189	6.18
0.7	80.0826 ± 1.5085	8.96
0.8	84.3155 ± 0.9986	10.76
0.9	90.9973 ± 0.9495	16.08
0.95	94.1750 ± 1.0631	23.22
0.96	94.8829 ± 1.4433	26.86
0.97	95.9627 ± 1.1626	32.80
0.98	96.6041 ± 1.5840	31.46
0.99	**96.8652 ± 1.1135**	**87.06**
1.0	96.7436 ± 1.2644	134.50

The figures in Table 5 tell us that the EM-ELM based feature selection algorithm has got its best performance of 97.4758% classification accuracy when the threshold is 0.99, that means when the minimum error is 0.01. The model can be obtained in around 157 seconds training time.

Table 5. Results of EM-ELM based feature selection algorithm.

Threshold	#selected features	Accuracy/%	Training time/s
0.5	10.6	82.1289±2.6502	4.3531
0.6	12.8	82.7246±4.1622	34.7938
0.7	20.8	80.4221±3.7150	34.9594
0.8	25.8	85.4944±2.5334	43.2781
0.9	23.8	90.2497±3.2873	102.4469
0.95	28.4	93.3608±4.0238	108.7563
0.98	27.8	96.3647±2.3314	128.1375
0.99	**27.6**	**97.4758±1.5545**	**157.3250**
1	28.6	94.9665±1.2675	193.7313

It can be seen from the results in Table 6 that the EM-ELM based feature selection algorithm can find the feature subset without losing the classification accuracy of EM-ELM but improving it in most cases among 5-fold cross validation experiments. So EM-ELM based feature selection algorithm can find the feature subset which can help medicine doctor to make proper diagnosis to the patients of erythemato-squamous diseases.

Table 6. Comparison between EM-ELM based feature selection and EM-ELM.

| | EM-ELM + improved F-score | | | EM-ELM | |
folds	#features	Accuracy/%	Training time/s	#features	Accuracy/%
fold1	29	**98.6486**	165.2813	34	95.9730
fold2	25	**95.8333**	138.1250	34	95.6111
fold3	27	**98.6111**	166.4844	34	98.0278
fold4	26	95.7143	148.7813	34	**96.7429**
fold5	31	**98.5714**	167.9531	34	97.9714
mean	27.6	**97.4758**	157.3250	34	96.8652

The results in Table 7 tell us that features 1, 18 and 32 were not selected into any feature subset in 5-fold cross validation experiments, which is coincident with ELM based feature selection algorithm. This fact demonstrates that these three features are indeed not significant to distinguish any specific erythemato-squamous disease.

Table 7. Feature subset by EM-ELM based feature selection algorithm.

folds	Feature subset
fold1	2,3,4,5,6,7,8,9,10,11,12,14,15,16,19,20,21,22,23,24,25,26,27,28,29,30,31,33,34
fold2	3,5,6,7,8,9,10,12,14,15,16,20,21,22,23,24,25,26,27,28,29,30,31,33,34
fold3	3,4,5,6 7,8,9,10,11,12,14,15,16,20,21,22,23,24,25,26,27,28,29,30,31,33,34
fold4	3,4,5,6,7,8,9,10,12,14,15,16,20,21,22,23,24,25,26,27,28,29,30,31,33,34
fold5	2,3,4,5,6,7,8,9,10,11,12,13,14,15,16,17,19,20,21,22,23,24,25,26,27,28,29,30,31,33,34

K-ELM Based Feature Selection Algorithm. The RBF is adopted as activation function in K-ELM, so the two parameters, including the penalty parameter C and the kernel parameter γ, must be determined. We adopt grid search technique with 5-fold cross-validation technique to find the best pair of parameters on the train subset. The penalty parameter C lies in the interval of $log_2C \in [-5, 15]$, and the kernel parameter γ is in the interval of $log_2\gamma \in [-15, 5]$. The parameter pair leading to the highest accuracy on the train subset will be found. After that we conduct 10-fold cross validation experiment with the best parameter pair on the train subset to detect the feature subset on which to build the K-ELM classifier. As the other two feature selection algorithms in this paper, the 5-fold cross validation experiments are conducted on the whole dataset. Table 8 lists the results of K-ELM based feature selection algorithm and that without feature selection process. Table 9 is the feature subset selected by K-ELM based feature selection algorithm in 5-fold cross validation experiments.

Table 8. Comparison between K-ELM based feature selection and K-ELM.

| | K-ELM + improved F-score | | | K-ELM | |
folds	#features	Accuracy/%	Training time/s	#features	Accuracy/%
fold1	24	**100.0000**	14.2031	34	97.2973
fold2	22	**97.2222**	13.7969	34	95.8333
fold3	23	**98.6111**	13.2969	34	98.6111
fold4	28	**97.1429**	13.5625	34	97.1429
fold5	24	97.1429	13.0156	34	**100.0000**
mean	24.2	**98.0238**	13.5750	34	97.7769

From the results in Table 8, we can see that K-ELM based feature selection algorithm can find the feature subset with better recognition performance except for that on the fifth fold, where the less than 0.03 classification accuracy is lost with less than 10 features compared to that with the whole original features. The mean accuracy of K-ELM based feature selection algorithm in 5-fold cross validation experiments is better than that of original K-ELM without feature selection. So we can say that feature selection is necessary.

Table 9. Feature subset by K-ELM based feature selection algorithm.

folds	Feature subset
fold1	5,6,7,8,9,10,12,14,15,16,20,21,22,23,24,25,26,27,28,29,30,31,33,34
fold2	5,6,7,8,9,10,12,14,15,16,20,21,22,24,25,26,27,28,29,30,31,33
fold3	5,6,7,8,9,10,12,14,15,16,20,21,22,24,25,26,27,28,29,30,31,33,34
fold4	2,3,4,5,6,7,8,9,10,12,14,15,16,19,20,21,22,23,24,25,26,27,28,29,30,31,33,34
fold5	4,5,6,7,8,9,10,12,14,15,16,20,21,22,24,25,26,27,28,29,30,31,33,34

Table 9 tells us that features 1, 11, 13, 17, 18 and 32 were not selected into any feature subset in 5-fold cross validation experiments, which include features not selected by ELM and EM-ELM based feature selection algorithms. The common unselected features by ELM, EM-ELM and K-ELM based feature selection algorithms are features 1, 18 and 32. This discloses that these three features are most insignificant to distinguish any specific erythemato-squamous disease, then the feature 17 followed by 11 and 13 are also insignificant features to recognize patients of erythemato-squamous diseases.

The Ensemble Diagnosis Model For erythemato-Squamous Disease.
This subsection will construct an ensemble diagnosis model for erythemato-squamous diseases by combing the diagnosis results of ELM, EM-ELM and K-ELM based feature selection algorithms for a patient via the majority voting technique, so as to obtain a much more proper diagnosis result. The ensemble idea is shown in Fig. 2. Table 10 gives the results of 5-fold cross validation experiments of the ensemble diagnosis model for erythemato-squamous diseases and that of its baseline classifiers.

Table 10. Accuracy of ensemble model of 5-fold cross validation experiments/%.

folds	ELM	EM-ELM	K-ELM	Ensemble model
fold1	98.6486	98.6486	100.0000	**100.0000**
fold2	97.2222	95.8333	97.2222	**97.2222**
fold3	97.2222	98.6111	98.6111	**98.6111**
fold4	97.1429	95.7143	97.1429	**97.1429**
fold5	98.5714	98.5714	97.1429	**98.5714**
Mean	97.7615	97.4758	98.0238	**98.3095**

From the results in Table 10, we can say that ensemble diagnosis model has got the best accuracy which is due to that it ensembles three base classifiers of ELM, EM-ELM, K-ELM built on their selected feature subsets respectively. K-ELM based feature selection algorithm is the best one among three feature selection algorithms proposed in this paper, and it can detect the feature subset on which a comparable classifier can be built.

3.3   The Comparison with Other Studies

This subsection will give the performance comparison between the algorithms proposed in this paper and the available ones for diagnosing erythemato-squamous diseases. Table 11 displays the performance comparison between the study in this paper and the available ones.

From the comparison in Table 11, we can see that our proposed algorithms have got the comparable performance in diagnosing erythema-squamous diseases compared to the available ones.

Table 11. Comparison between available studies for erythemato-squamous diseases

Authors	Algorithms	Accuracy/%
Übeyli and Güler (2005) [22]	ANFIS	95.50
Luukka and Leppälampi (2006) [12]	Fuzzy similarity-based classification	97.02
Polat and Günes (2006) [17]	Fuzzy weighted pre-processing	88.18
	K-NN based weighted pre-processing	97.57
	Decision tree	99.00
Nanni (2006) [13]	LSVM	97.22
	RS	97.22
	B1_5	97.50
	B1_10	98.10
	B1_15	97.22
	B2_5	97.50
	B2_10	97.80
	B2_15	98.30
Luukka (2007) [11]	Similarity measure	97.80
Übeyli (2008) [19]	Multiclass SVM with the ECOC	98.32
Polat and Günes (2009) [18]	C4.5 and one-against-all	96.71
Übeylii (2009) [20]	CNN	97.77
Liu et al. (2009) [9]	Naïve Bayes	96.72
	1-NN	92.18
	C4.5	95.08
	PIPPER	92.20
Karabatak and Ince (2009) [8]	AR and NN	98.61
Übeyli and Doğdu (2010) [21]	K-means clustering	94.22
Xie et al. (2011) [28]	IFSFS+SVM	98.61
Xie et al. (2012) [25]	GFSFS+SVM	98.89
	modified GFSFS+SVM	99.17
	GFSFFS+SVM	96.08
	modified GFSFFS+SVM	98.33
	GFSBFS+SVM	95.81
	modified GFSBFS+SVM	95.28
Xie et al. (2013) [26]	two-stage GFSFS	100
	two-stage new GFSFS	100
	two-stage GFSFFS	100
	two-stage new GFSFFS	100
	two-stage GFSBFS	100
	two-stage new GFSBFS	97.06
Özcift and Gülten (2013) [14]	GA+BN	99.20
Abdi and Giveki (2013) [1]	PSO+SVM	98.91
Liu et al (2015) [10]	mRMR+K-ELM	98.55
Wang and Xie (2017) [23]	GrC+SVM	98.61
This study	improved F-score+ELM	97.7615
	improved F-score+EM-ELM	97.4758
	improved F-score+K-LEM	98.0238
	Ensemble model	98.3095

4   Conclusions and Future Works

Three feature selection algorithms and one ensemble diagnosis model were proposed in this paper for diagnosing erythemato-squamous diseases. The experimental results demonstrate that the proposed algorithms are comparable to the available ones. However, ELM and EM-ELM are unstable learning machines whose accuracies are affected by their random weights and thresholds. How to improve the stable of ELM and EM-ELM based features selection algorithms need further studying.

References

1. Abdi, M.J., Giveki, D.: Automatic detection of erythemato-squamous diseases using PSO-SVM based on association rules. Eng. Appl. Artif. Intell. **26**(1), 603–608 (2013)
2. Dheeru, D., Karra Taniskidou, E.: UCI machine learning repository (2017). http://archive.ics.uci.edu/ml
3. Ding, C., Peng, H.: Minimum redundancy feature selection from microarray gene expression data. J. Bioinform. Comput. Biol. **3**(02), 185–205 (2005)
4. Feng, G., Huang, G., Lin, Q., Gay, R.K.L.: Error minimized extreme learning machine with growth of hidden nodes and incremental learning. IEEE Trans. Neural Netw. **20**(8), 1352–1357 (2009)
5. Huang, G., Zhou, H., Ding, X., Zhang, R.: Extreme learning machine for regression and multiclass classification. IEEE Trans. Syst., Man, Cybern. Part B (Cybern.) **42**(2), 513–529 (2012)
6. Huang, G., Zhu, Q., Siew, C.K.: Extreme learning machine: theory and applications. Neurocomputing **70**(1–3), 489–501 (2006)
7. Kabir, E., Siuly, S., Cao, J., Wang, H.: A computer aided analysis scheme for detecting epileptic seizure from EEG data. Int. J. Comput. Intell. Syst. **11**, 663–671 (2018)
8. Karabatak, M., Ince, M.C.: A new feature selection method based on association rules for diagnosis of erythemato-squamous diseases. Expert. Syst. Appl. **36**(10), 12500–12505 (2009)
9. Liu, H., Sun, J., Liu, L., Zhang, H.: Feature selection with dynamic mutual information. Pattern Recogn. **42**(7), 1330–1339 (2009)
10. Liu, T., Hu, L., Ma, C., Wang, Z.Y., Chen, H.L.: A fast approach for detection of erythemato-squamous diseases based on extreme learning machine with maximum relevance minimum redundancy feature selection. Int. J. Syst. Sci. **46**(5), 919–931 (2015)
11. Luukka, P.: Similarity classifier using similarity measure derived from Yu's norms in classification of medical data sets. Comput. Biol. Med. **37**(8), 1133–1140 (2007)
12. Luukka, P., Leppälampi, T.: Similarity classifier with generalized mean applied to medical data. Comput. Biol. Med. **36**(9), 1026–1040 (2006)
13. Nanni, L.: An ensemble of classifiers for the diagnosis of erythemato-squamous diseases. Neurocomputing **69**(7–9), 842–845 (2006)
14. Özcift, A., Gülten, A.: Genetic algorithm wrapped Bayesian network feature selection applied to differential diagnosis of erythemato-squamous diseases. Digit. Sig. Process. **23**(1), 230–237 (2013)

15. Peng, M., Xie, Q., Wang, H., Zhang, Y., Gang, T.: Bayesian sparse topical coding. IEEE Trans. Knowl. Data Eng. **30**, 1 (2018). https://doi.org/10.1109/TKDE.2018.2847707

16. Peng, M., et al.: Mining event-oriented topics in microblog stream with unsupervised multi-view hierarchical embedding. ACM Trans. Knowl. Discov. Data **20**(3), 38:1–38:26 (2018). https://doi.org/10.1145/3173044, http://doi.acm.org/10.1145/3173044

17. Polat, K., Güneş, S.: The effect to diagnostic accuracy of decision tree classifier of fuzzy and k-NN based weighted pre-processing methods to diagnosis of erythemato-squamous diseases. Digital Signal Process. **16**(6), 922–930 (2006)

18. Polat, K., Güneş, S.: A novel hybrid intelligent method based on c4.5 decision tree classifier and one-against-all approach for multi-class classification problems. Expert Syst. Appl. **36**(2), 1587–1592 (2009)

19. Übeyli, E.D.: Multiclass support vector machines for diagnosis of erythemato-squamous diseases. Expert Syst. Appl. **35**(8), 1733–1740 (2008)

20. Übeyli, E.D.: Combined neural networks for diagnosis of erythemato-squamous diseases. Expert Syst. Appl. **36**(3), 5107–5112 (2009)

21. Übeyli, E.D., Doğdu, E.: Automatic detection of erythemato-squamous diseases using k-means clustering. J. Med. Syst. **34**(2), 179–184 (2010)

22. Übeylı, E.D., Güler, I.: Automatic detection of erythemato-squamous diseases using adaptive neuro-fuzzy inference systems. Comput. Biol. Med. **35**(5), 421–433 (2005)

23. Wang, Y., Xie, J.: Granular computing combined with support vector machines for diagnosing erythemato-squamous diseases. In: Siuly, S., et al. (eds.) HIS 2017. LNCS, vol. 10594, pp. 56–68. Springer, Cham (2017). https://doi.org/10.1007/978-3-319-69182-4_7

24. Whitney, A.W.: A direct method of nonparametric measurement selection. IEEE Trans. Comput. **100**(9), 1100–1103 (1971)

25. Xie, J., Lei, J., Xie, W., Gao, X., Shi, Y., Liu, X.: Novel hybrid feature selection algorithms for diagnosing erythemato-squamous diseases. In: He, J., Liu, X., Krupinski, E.A., Xu, G. (eds.) HIS 2012. LNCS, vol. 7231, pp. 173–185. Springer, Heidelberg (2012). https://doi.org/10.1007/978-3-642-29361-0_21

26. Xie, J., Lei, J., Xie, W., Shi, Y., Liu, X.: Two-stage hybrid feature selection algorithms for diagnosing erythemato-squamous diseases. Health Inf. Sci. Syst. **1**(1), 10 (2013)

27. Xie, J., Li, Y., Zhou, Y., Wang, M.: Differential feature recognition of breast cancer patients based on minimum spanning tree clustering and F-statistics. In: Yin, X., Geller, J., Li, Y., Zhou, R., Wang, H., Zhang, Y. (eds.) HIS 2016. LNCS, vol. 10038, pp. 194–204. Springer, Cham (2016). https://doi.org/10.1007/978-3-319-48335-1_21

28. Xie, J., Wang, C.: Using support vector machines with a novel hybrid feature selection method for diagnosis of erythemato-squamous diseases. Expert Syst. Appl. **38**(5), 5809–5815 (2011)

29. Xie, J., Xie, W., Wang, C., Gao, X.: A novel hybrid feature selection method based on IFSFFS and SVM for the diagnosis of erythemato-squamous diseases. In: Proceedings of the First Workshop on Applications of Pattern Analysis, pp. 142–151 (2010)

Sentiment Classification with Medical Word Embeddings and Sequence Representation for Drug Reviews

Sisi Liu and Ickjai Lee[✉] [iD]

Discipline of Computer Science and Information Technology,
College of Science and Engineering, James Cook University,
PO Box 6811, Cairns, QLD 4870, Australia
sisi.liu@my.jcu.edu.au, ickjai.lee@jcu.edu.au

Abstract. Medical sentiments derived from health-care related documents, such as health reviews, tweets or forums, have been an indispensable resource for studying insights into patient health conditions and generating additional information for health professionals to provide more supportive treatments. However, approaches implemented in previous studies indicate inadequacy in discovering insights into review details and implicit emotional information due to domain specificities. We propose a sentiment classification framework with medical word embeddings and sequence representation for drug review datasets. Empirical results on different vector transformation methods imply the superiority of sequence incorporated medical sentiment lexicon using machine learning classifiers. Experiments on various word embeddings with convolutional neural network model further justify the effectiveness of medical sentiment word embeddings in sentiment classification for drug reviews.

1 Introduction

Sentiment analysis or opinion mining for text datasets in medical settings, such as drug reviews, clinical narratives or health forum comments, has been an appealing research area nowadays. For instance, [14] utilized machine learning techniques to build semi-automatic emotion annotation system for on-line health forums due to the low level agreements among human annotators; [1] conducted a study on sentiment analysis for medical forums using combined sentiment lexicon and supervised learning approaches; and [20] proposed a semantic-based supervised learning method for patient knowledge retrieval. These studies imply the potential usefulness of conducting sentiment analysis and related tasks on medical datasets. They generate subjective opinion information that not only benefits patients in gaining supports and knowledge from peers, but also provides health professionals with more adjusted and suitable prescriptions or treatments. Unlike conventional social media or product review datasets that contain relatively direct emotional expressions, health and medical domain related datasets are generally more implicit and massaged with medical terminology. Drug reviews, comparing with other types of health-care archives or medical documents, are

S. Siuly et al. (Eds.): HIS 2018, LNCS 11148, pp. 75–86, 2018.
https://doi.org/10.1007/978-3-030-01078-2_7

less sensitive in terms of private information and easier to retrieve the ground truth using review ratings [9]. Although a few opinion mining studies have been conducted on drug reviews, research limitations mainly reside in the lack of insights into review details and implicit emotional information due to domain specificities [6,8,9].

With the wide application of deep learning techniques to natural language analysis tasks, as well as inspired by a recent study conducted by [4] using word embeddings to generate vector representations for clinical concepts, this study aims at implementing word embedding techniques, and applying them to existing sentiment lexicon to develop a medical domain specific sentiment lexicon and sequence vector representation for better sentiment classification performance. Main contributions of this study are listed as below:

- proposing a technique for generating medical domain specific sentiment lexicon using word embeddings;
- incorporating the temporal sequence as a feature into the vector transformation process for sentiment classification;
- experimenting on four state-of-the-art machine learning algorithms, Support Vector Machine (SVM), Logistic Regression (LR), Multilayer Perceptron (MLP) and Radial Basis Function Neural Network (RBFNN), with various vector transformation methods using medical sentiment lexicon as a feature;
- evaluating medical sentiment lexicon embeddings against other pre-trained word embeddings, such as Word2Vec [15] and Global Vectors (GloVe) [17], on Convolutional Neural Network (CNN) model.

2   Related Work

Medical sentiment analysis is an extension to traditional sentiment analysis aiming at extracting sentiments from medical documents. Applying sentiment analysis to text documents in medical settings has a potential for providing mutual benefits for both health-care professionals and patients regarding the outcomes of medical treatments and causes of positive and negative medical conditions [1,2,6]. In terms of content and linguistic peculiarities, opinion mining or sentiment analysis for medical documents is expected to involve domain-specific sentiment sources [6].

Implementation of sentiment lexicon has been a popular approach in various research on sentiment analysis or opinion mining for medical documents. For example, [1] applied a subjectivity lexicon with supervised learning approaches for discovering sentiments from hearing loss forums, and [16] proposed a hybrid approach incorporating the WordNet of medical events for conducting sentiment extraction from medical contexts. Among sentiment lexicons that are publicly available, SentiWordNet (SWN) [3] is the one that covers a wide range of sentiment phrases with a semi-supervised labeling approach. Even though some issues with applications of SWN lexicon in medical settings are observed from previous studies including inferior performance, influence of noise features, and lack of domain knowledge [1,2,6,16], SWN has been studied and implemented for sentiment analysis and its related tasks in recent research [21]. To better utilize SWN lexicon as a feature extraction method for medical sentiment analysis tasks and to improve its performance, a question on how to handle the above mentioned issues remains to be solved.

As a robust feature learning and topic modeling technique, word embedding achieves good performance in text mining and natural language processing tasks. Some studies have been conducted on the implementation of medical domain knowledge into biomedical natural language processing using word embedding techniques. For instance, [4] proposed an approach named *cui2vec* to generate word embeddings for medical concepts with a trained corpus of 20 million clinical notes and 1.7 million biomedical journal articles; [10] incorporated text mining techniques, such as stem and chunk, to train domain-specific word embeddings for biomedical texts; and [12] implemented word embeddings with n-gram model for biological event extraction from texts. However, as these studies mainly focus on the application of word embeddings to medical concepts rather than medical related sentiment phrases, it is improper to directly apply techniques derived from these studies to extracting sentiment from health-care documents.

3   Sentiment Classification with Medical Word Embeddings and Sequence Representation

A brief flow work of the proposed method that incorporates text preprocessing, vector transformation and sentiment classification is presented in Fig. 1. Vector transformation process is subdivided into medical word embedding for SWN and sequence in feature representation. To maintain the integrity of drug review documents, text cleaning is conducted at a minimal level during preprocessing step considering the concept of word embedding and sentiment sequence is less sensitive to noise than other traditional feature transformation techniques. Details will be discussed in the following subsections.

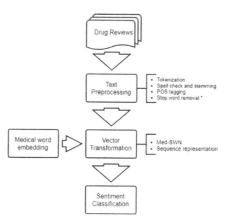

Fig. 1. Overall framework of proposed sentiment classification with medical word embeddings and sequence representation.

Let $\mathcal{DR}$ denote a collection of drug reviews containing review documents $dr_1, dr_2, \ldots, dr_i$, and $\mathcal{T}$ denote a set of post-processed word list in each review document containing tokens $t_1, t_2, \ldots, t_j$. A detailed pseudo code for review data preprocessing is described in Pseudocode 1. To highlight, the open source NLP toolkit developed by Apache Lucene [5] is utilized to implement tokenization (*tokenize()*), spell check (*SpellChecker()*), stemming (*stem()*), and Part-of-Speech (POS) tagging(*tag()*) functions for data cleaning purpose. Note that, a stop word removal, implemented using *stopAnalyzer()* and *ENGLISH_STOP_WORD_LIST* developed by Stanford NLP packages [13], is not applied for the sequence incorporated feature representation as removing phrases influences the chronological order of the sentiment expressed in a review document.

Pseudocode 1. TextPreprocessing

1: **Input:** A set of review documents $\mathcal{DR}$ with labels $\mathcal{L}$.
2: **Output:** Each review document $dr_i \in \mathcal{DR}$ represented with a collection of tokens t_n in a refined word list $\mathcal{T}$.
3: **for** each review document $dr_i \in \mathcal{DR}$ **do**
4:     Tokenize dr_i using *tokenize()* function;
5:     **for** each token $t_j \in \mathcal{T}$ **do**
6:         Apply spell check using *SpellChecker()* object;
7:         Stem t_j using *stem()* function;
8:         **if** $t_j \in ENGLISH\_STOP\_WORD\_LIST$ **then**
9:             Remove t_j from $\mathcal{T}$;
10:            Generate POS tags to t_j using *tagger()* function;
11:            Return each document dr_i with a list of refined words $\mathcal{T}$;
12:        **end if**
13:    **end for**
14: **end for**

3.1   Vector Transformation

Vector transformation is a process to convert a text document into an array of numeric vectors that could be compiled by machine learning algorithms. As discussed previously, although SWN is a well-structured and refined sentiment lexicon with more than $140,000$ semi-supervised labeled sentiment phrases, it is not developed to suit for medical domain knowledge. Thus, a self-trained word embeddings on large clinical narrative corpus is generated to enlarge the original SWN with more health-care related sentiment phrases. To obtain sentiment sequence information, each review document is transformed into a chronologically ordered set of sentiment phrases represented with their corresponding values in this expanded SWN.

Medical Word Embedding for SWN Lexicon. SWN 3.0 [3] serves as the foundation for generating sentiment features in this study. Denote $\mathcal{SWN}$ as a set of sentiment phrases $\mathcal{SP} = \{sp_1, sp_2, \ldots, sp_n\}$, and each sentiment phrase sp_i contains a set of synset terms $\mathcal{ST} = \{st_1, st_2, \ldots, st_m\}$ annotated with a pos_j score, a neg_j score and a ranking value w_j. Denote a set of sentiment values $\mathcal{V} = \{v_1, v_2, \ldots, v_n\}$ associated with sentiment phrases, each sentiment value is calculated by the weighted average subject score $subj$ of all synset terms belonging to the sentiment phrase. Equation 1 describes the calculation for subject score $subj$ for each synset term st_j of a sentiment phrase sp_i and its corresponding sentiment value v_i.

$$subj = pos_j - neg_j, \; for \; j \in \mathcal{ST},$$
$$v_i = \frac{\sum_{i=1}^{j} w_i subj_i}{\sum_{i=1}^{j} w_i}, \; for \; i \in \mathcal{SP} \; and \; j \in \mathcal{ST}. \tag{1}$$

Medical documents are rarely open-source and publicly available due to the sensitivity and privacy concern. MIMIC II [19], Multi-parameter Intelligent Monitoring for Intensive Care, is an archived database containing patient records generated from over 800 ICU patients. This database is shared for scientific research, and also it includes clinical text documents, such as medical history records, radiology reports, and nursing notes, which have similar types and formats to the drug review dataset used for this study. Research conducted by [7] suggests that comparing to other types of medical documents, radiology reports and nursing notes is involved in relatively more emotional expressions and sentiments. With adequate file processing steps, a corpus of 3,958 clinical documents is fed into a *word2vec* model generated by *gensim*, a well-developed open-source Python topic and vector space modeling library [18]. Post-trained word embeddings of this corpus are stored for further process. Meanwhile, a trained medical *word2vec* model is implemented for discovering similar terms of sentiment phrases in SWN. Given a specific sentiment phrase, we compute the cosine similarity using *word2vec*. If any returned association term is not in the existing SWN, we compute the sentiment value by multiplying a similarity value with the corresponding sentiment value of specific sentiment phrases in SWN. The mathematical equation of cosine similarity between two sentiment phase vectors, v and w, is defined as follows:

$$cos\_sim(v, w) = \frac{v \cdot w}{\|v\| \|w\|} = \frac{\sum_i^n v_i \times w_i}{\sqrt{\sum_i^n v_i^2} \times \sqrt{\sum_i^n w_i^2}}. \tag{2}$$

To be more specific, Pseudocode 2 summarizes the computational process for generating medical sentiment lexicon using *word2vec* model. Denote $\mathcal{CN}$ as a collection of clinical narratives containing clinical documents $\{cn_1, cn_2, \ldots, cn_k\}$, T_{cn} as a set of post-processed word list in each clinical documents. Train T_{cn} with $Word2Vec()$ object using *gensim* library. After achieving a post-trained *word2vec* model, we compute the cosine similarity measurement of each sentiment phrase sp_i with vocabulary of the model. Denote $\mathcal{MT} = \{mt_1, mt_2, \ldots, mt_l\}$ as a set of terms returned from the cosine similarity measurement of sentiment phrase sp_i that exists in the drug review corpus $\mathcal{DR}$,

---

Pseudocode 2. AlgoMed-SWN

1: **Input:** A collection of review documents $\mathcal{DR}$, clinical documents $\mathcal{CN}$, and $\mathcal{SWN}$
   lexicon with sentiment phrases sp_n and values v_n.
2: **Output:** $Med-SWN$ with a list of sentiment phrases msp_t with word embeddings
   and values $vmed_t$.
3: **for** each clinical document cn_k in clinical narrative corpus $\mathcal{CN}$ **do**
4:      Tokenize each document cn_k and remove non alpha-numeric value;
5:      Return a set of post-processed token list T_{cn};
6: **end for**
7: Train T_{cn} with $Word2Vec()$ model;
8: Return $medicalword2vec$ model and store word embeddings;
9: **for** each sentiment phrase sp_n **do**
10:     Compile $cos\_sim()$ function;
11:     **for** each term $mt_l \in \mathcal{DR}$ **do**
12:         Store mt_l as msp_t into $Med-SWN$;
13:         Compute $cos\_sim() * v_n$ as sentiment value $vmed_t$ for $vmed_t$;
14:     **end for**
15: **end for**
16: **for** each $msp_t \in Med-SWN$ **do**
17:     Use $medicalword2vec$ model to generate word embeddings for msp_t;
18: **end for**

$Med-SWN$ as a new list of sentiment phrases $\{msp_1, msp_2, \ldots, msp_t\}$ including terms generated from $word2vec$ model, and $V_{med} = \{vmed_1, vmed_2, \ldots, vmed_t\}$ as a list of sentiment values associated with the sentiment phrases. The sentiment value of a new sentiment phrase msp_t is calculated by the multiplication of cosine similarity value with v_i and stored in $Med-SWN$ as $vmed_t$. Finally, we use the $word2vec$ model trained using $\mathcal{CN}$ to generate word embeddings for each sentiment phrase msp_t in $Med-SWN$ and store them for future experiments.

Sequence in Feature Representation. As drug reviews are variable in length, frequency or term-weighted feature representation approaches are suitable and adequate. Considering sequence in feature representation is one direction of solving this variable length issue. For instance, [14] enriched a sequential pattern algorithm during the sentence labeling process. The concept of incorporating sentiment sequence information into document-based sentiment analysis is achieved through extracting Med-SWN features in a chronological order.

As pointed out earlier, no stop word removal is to be performed for sequence incorporated feature representation as the idea of keeping a chronological order of sentiment feature in a document ensures the integrity of the document. A sample drug review in the final vector representation is illustrated as follows, in which *position* represents the nth slot of a sentiment phrase in each review document and v represents the corresponding sentiment value of the word Med-SWN lexicon returns. For instance, given a sentence 'I like the dress you brought yesterday', a term *'like'* is represented as *'2: 0.38'* after converting this sentence into vector representation. In contrast, performing stop word removal changes the term *'like'* into the first position.

$$< id \quad label \quad position_1: \quad v_1 \quad position_2: \quad v_2 \quad \ldots \quad position_n: \quad v_n >$$

3.2   Sentiment Classification

Our sentiment classification process includes two sets of experiments on the comparison of sentiment classification results: (a) different vector representation methods using sentiment lexicon with various machine learning algorithms; (b) self-trained medical sentiment lexicon over other pre-trained word embeddings, including Word2Vec and GloVe. Empirical results for the former are evaluated using the confusion matrix (*precision, recall* and *f−measure*), and for the latter are evaluated using classification accuracy. Both evaluations are conducted using the 10-fold cross validation.

Four state-of-the-art machine learning algorithms, including SVM, LR, MLP and RBFNN, are evaluated for the performance of classification results with different vector representation methods. Algorithms are all implemented using library packages pre-developed by WEKA (https://www.cs.waikato.ac.nz/ml/weka/) with adjusted parameter settings for optimal outcomes. Among the four algorithms above, SVM and RBFNN are evaluated for outstanding performance in medical sentiment classification tasks, whilst LR and MLP are introduced as referential algorithms for the logistic supervised learning approach and neural network model, respectively. With similar settings as described in [14,16], SVM represents the algorithm wrapped by Sequential Minimal Optimization (SMO) with the RBF kernel as a hyperplane for separating non linearly separable instances. RBFNN is utilized due to its superior performance for classifying sentiments for drug reviews in [9]. RBFNN is a three layer neural network with one input layer and one output layer scaled by a hidden non-linear RBF layer, in which the hidden layer is composed of neurons weighted by Gaussian radial basis function and concatenated using Euclidean distance [22]. Since both SVM and RBFNN utilize the RBF kernel, the mathematical equation is concluded as follows, in which $\exp\left[-\delta\|x-a_i\|^2\right]$ denotes a Gaussian basis function computing the distance of an instance to its center vector with an approximation function δ and an optimization function n_i:

$$RBF(x) = \sum_{i=1}^{N} n_i \exp\left[-\delta\|x-c_i\|^2\right]. \tag{3}$$

Performance of classification models is evaluated using confusion matrix including *precision, recall* and *f − measure*, in which *precision* is defined by the number of true positive instances over the number of classified positive instances; *recall* is defined by the number of true positive instances over the number of real positive instances; and *f − measure* is defined by the weighted average of precision and true positive rate (*recall*).

Once a post-trained *word2vec* model using clinical narrative corpus is obtained, a test against other pre-trained word embeddings is conducted using CNN model, a refined neural network model widely adopted for natural language processing and its related tasks [11, 12]. Word2Vec [15], and GloVe are the pretrained word embedding options for comparative results against n-gram, medical SWN word embeddings to prove the feasibility of classification performance with domain specific knowledge. Evaluation criterion is a sole accuracy. Word2Vec implemented for comparative experiments is a pre-trained word embeddings of 300 dimensions on Google news corpus with around 3 billion running words, originated from https://code.google.com/archive/p/word2vec/. GloVe refers to a collection of word embeddings with 50 dimensions trained on aggregated statistics of global word co-occurrence with a vocabulary of 6 billion [17].

4   Empirical Results and Discussions

4.1   Dataset

In this study, a mixed dataset of 500 drug reviews containing 247 negative and 253 positive drug reviews from two sources is generated for the purpose of testing the proposed method across different review sources to avoid the unanimity and duplication of reviews. As discussed in [9], it is suspected that drug reviews occasionally intermix with comments on side effects. To test whether the above mentioned observation would affect the performance of sentiment classification, we intentionally introduce a comment on side effects dataset into the drug review dataset for experiments. We expect this introduction will complicate the classification task and negatively affect the classification accuracy.

A set of 253 positive reviews is extracted from a public drug review website available at https://www.askapatient.com/. Reviews are manually selected from drugs that have average ratings higher than 3.0 with scores of 4.0 or 5.0 out of 5.0. Due to the fact that drug reactions varied from person to person, judging reviews selected from drugs with an average score of 3.0 as positive is to minimize the chance of invalid reviews. A set of 247 negative reviews is generated using the annotated training adverse drug reaction (ADR) review dataset [23]. Since all reviews are stated with ADR, it is reasonable to convert annotations into negative labels.

Sample positive and negative reviews are depicted as follows:

```
P: I get a good sleep. It helps with colds. I use it as needed
and feel no rebound effect when I don't take it. I have also
discovered that it helps my acid reflux, which I developed from
taking anti inflammatory medication for arthritis.
N: horrible joint pain, insomnia, hot flashes, anxiety, hair
not growing, brain not working well.
```

4.2   Medical Word Embeddings and Med-SWN

As stated in previous section, the initial SWN contains more than 140,000 sentiment phrases, which is extremely computation intensive. Therefore, before expanding the SWN, a pruning process to remove those phrases with no occurrence in any drug review document is performed, and as a result a pruned SWN lexicon containing 1,608 phrases is created.

Performance of *word2vec* model is greatly influenced by parameter settings. With a few attempts, the final medical word embeddings are generated using skip-gram framework with an embedding size of 100, a window size of 5, a minimum word count of 50 in order to optimize experimental results. Final embedding is performed on a corpus with a vocabulary of 86,547.

Table 1. Sample sentiment phrases generated from Med-SWN.

Original SWN Phrase	Value	Expanded SWN Phrase	Value
Nervous	−0.1149	Frustrating	−0.0844
Scratch	−0.0459	Scabs	−0.0392
Swollen	−0.75	Bruise	−0.526
Poison	−0.125	Sprays	−0.0843
Poor	−0.4849	Impairment	−0.1768
Prefer	0.48	Willing	0.3291
Hope	0.0892	Meaning	0.0171

Table 1 illustrates some sample opinion words from medical SWN. The left two columns indicate the sentiment phrases and their corresponding values in the original SWN and the right two columns are the new sentiment terms generated from the original ones. Results indicate an additional 769 sentiment terms discovered using medical word embeddings incorporated SWN, which is approximately 47.8% increase of the original lexicon, implying that drug reviews do contain medical domain specific information that is missed out with the general sentiment lexicon.

4.3   Sentiment Classification Results and Discussions

In terms of sentiment classification for different vector representations experiments, final parameter settings for four machine learning algorithms are as follows: SVM results are achieved with a complexity parameter c set to 5; LR and RBFNN results are achieved using default settings; and MLP results are achieved with 3 hidden layers and a batch size of 100.

Table 2 illustrates classification results of four machine learning algorithms using different vector representations where bold texts indicate those to be highlighted. Results epitomize that vector transformation methods with sequence incorporated Med-SWN lexicon achieve the highest precision of 0.598 over other three methods. Although the highest $f - measure$ of 0.584 among all test results is achieved with the sequence incorporated SWN lexicon vector representation, two other machine learning algorithms (SVM and RBFNN) have better $f - measure$ with the sequence incorporated Med-SWN. In conclusion, sequence incorporated vector representation methods produce better results than those without sequence, and the enhanced SWN lexicon with medical embeddings has a potential to improve performance as well.

Table 2. Evaluation results of different vector representations of four supervised learning algorithms (P: Precision; R: Recall; F: $f - measure$).

	SWN			Med-SWN			Seq-SWN			Seq-MSWN		
	P	R	F	P	R	F	P	R	F	P	R	F
SVM	0.517	0.514	0.515	0.535	0.52	0.527	0.549	0.54	0.544	0.556	0.548	**0.552**
LR	0.511	0.512	0.511	0.535	0.52	0.527	0.555	0.54	**0.547**	0.536	0.534	0.534
MLP	0.509	0.505	0.507	0.521	0.52	0.520	0.586	0.582	**0.584**	0.548	0.546	0.547
RBFNN	0.571	0.546	0.558	0.568	0.544	0.556	0.589	0.56	0.574	**0.598**	0.566	**0.581**

Table 3. Evaluation of various word embeddings using CNN model.

Parameter settings	Value	Word Embeddings	Accuracy
Filter window size	[3,4,5]	n-gram	0.5375
Number of filters	128	GloVe	0.5225
Dropout probability	0.5	Word2Vec	0.655
Batch size	64	SWNVec	0.525
Epochs	100	MedVec	0.5875
		Med-SWNVec	**0.6975**

To further justify the effectiveness and feasibility of medical sentiment lexicon, a test on comparison among different word embeddings is conducted using CNN model. Table 3 describes the parameter settings for CNN model as well as the classification accuracy under different word embeddings. Results indicate that word embeddings with Med-SWN lexicon are able to achieve a slightly higher accuracy score of 0.6975 when compared to other types of word embeddings. However, considering the size of the dataset, models established by CNN with word embeddings as input features are trained with limitations. Hence, further experiments are required to draw a solid conclusion.

5   Conclusion

In this study, drug review datasets are utilized for empirical experiments on the feasibility and effectiveness of medical sentiment word embeddings with sequence representation for sentiment classification in medical settings. To minimize the influence of different textual features for vector transformation, SWN lexicon is selected as the sole base sentiment features. With medical sentiment features extracted using word embeddings, experimental results demonstrate that the sequence incorporated vector transformation is proven to outperform conventional frequency or term weighting based vector transformation techniques. In addition, evaluations on various word embeddings justify the effectiveness of medical sentiment word embeddings in sentiment classification tasks for health documents.

Even though empirical experiments support the feasibility and superiority of the proposed method in learning insights into drug reviews and extracting sentiments, overall performance exhibits there is a space for improvements. Since there are no public medical text datasets with ground truth values for sentiment benchmark, this study is limited to test the comprehensive feasibility and effectiveness of sentiment word embeddings in medical contexts. This study manually captures a dataset with two different data sources considering the availability of datasets: positive reviews based on comments whilst negative reviews based on side effects. This disparity might have negatively affected classification accuracies. Future research directions are in two folds. First, generating more balanced and larger benchmark datasets with ground truth for comparative studies. Second, future studies need to experiment the proposed framework with larger and various datasets to confirm the feasibility and effectiveness of the proposed method.

References

1. Ali, T., Schramm, D., Sokolova, M., Inkpen, D.: Can i hear you? Sentiment analysis on medical forums. In: Proceedings of the Sixth International Joint Conference on Natural Language Processing, pp. 667–673 (2013)
2. Asghar, M.Z., et al.: Medical opinion lexicon: an incremental model for mining health reviews. Int. J. Acad. Res. **6**(1), 295–302 (2014)
3. Baccianella, S., Esuli, A., Sebastiani, F.: SentiWordNet 3.0: an enhanced lexical resource for sentiment analysis and opinion mining. In: LREC, vol. 10, pp. 2200–2204 (2010)
4. Beam, A.L., et al.: Clinical concept embeddings learned from massive sources of medical data. arXiv preprint arXiv:1804.01486 (2018)
5. Białecki, A., Muir, R., Ingersoll, G., Imagination, L.: Apache Lucene 4. In: SIGIR 2012 workshop on open source information retrieval, p. 17 (2012)
6. Denecke, K., Deng, Y.: Sentiment analysis in medical settings: new opportunities and challenges. Artif. Intell. Med. **64**(1), 17–27 (2015)
7. Deng, Y., Stoehr, M., Denecke, K.: Retrieving attitudes: Sentiment analysis from clinical narratives. In: MedIR@ SIGIR, pp. 12–15 (2014)
8. Gohil, S., Vuik, S., Darzi, A.: Sentiment analysis of health care tweets: review of the methods used. JMIR Public Health Surveill. **4**(2), e43 (2018)
9. Gopalakrishnan, V., Ramaswamy, C.: Patient opinion mining to analyze drugs satisfaction using supervised learning. J. Appl. Res. Technol. **15**(4), 311–319 (2017)

10. Jiang, Z., Li, L., Huang, D., Jin, L.: Training word embeddings for deep learning in biomedical text mining tasks. In: 2015 IEEE International Conference on Bioinformatics and Biomedicine (BIBM), pp. 625–628. IEEE (2015)
11. Kim, Y.: Convolutional neural networks for sentence classification. arXiv preprint arXiv:1408.5882 (2014)
12. Li, C., Song, R., Liakata, M., Vlachos, A., Seneff, S., Zhang, X.: Using word embedding for bio-event extraction. Proc. BioNLP **15**, 121–126 (2015)
13. Manning, C., Surdeanu, M., Bauer, J., Finkel, J., Bethard, S., McClosky, D.: The Stanford coreNLP natural language processing toolkit. In: Proceedings of 52nd Annual Meeting of the Association for Computational Linguistics: System Demonstrations, pp. 55–60 (2014)
14. Melzi, S., Abdaoui, A., Azé, J., Bringay, S., Poncelet, P., Galtier, F.: Patient's rationale: Patient knowledge retrieval from health forums. In: eTELEMED: eHealth, Telemedicine, and Social Medicine (2014)
15. Mikolov, T., Chen, K., Corrado, G., Dean, J.: Efficient estimation of word representations in vector space. arXiv preprint arXiv:1301.3781 (2013)
16. Mondal, A., Satapathy, R., Das, D., Bandyopadhyay, S.: A hybrid approach based sentiment extraction from medical context. In: SAAIP@ IJCAI, vol. 1619, pp. 35–40 (2016)
17. Pennington, J., Socher, R., Manning, C.: Glove: Global vectors for word representation. In: Proceedings of the 2014 Conference on Empirical Methods in Natural Language Processing (EMNLP), pp. 1532–1543 (2014)
18. Rehurek, R., Sojka, P.: Software framework for topic modelling with large corpora. In: Proceedings of the LREC 2010 Workshop on New Challenges for NLP Frameworks. Citeseer (2010)
19. Saeed, M., Lieu, C., Raber, G., Mark, R.G.: Mimic ii: a massive temporal ICU patient database to support research in intelligent patient monitoring. In: Computers in Cardiology, 2002, pp. 641–644. IEEE (2002)
20. Salas-Zárate, M.D.P., et al.: Sentiment analysis on tweets about diabetes: an aspect-level approach. In: Computational and Mathematical Methods in Medicine 2017 (2017)
21. Sarawgi, K., Pathak, V.: Opinion mining: aspect level sentiment analysis using SentiWordNet and Amazon web services. Int. J. Comput. Appl. **158**(6) (2017)
22. Scholkopf, B., et al.: Comparing support vector machines with Gaussian kernels to radial basis function classifiers. IEEE Trans. Signal Process. **45**(11), 2758–2765 (1997)
23. Yates, A., Goharian, N.: ADRTrace: detecting expected and unexpected adverse drug reactions from user reviews on social media sites. In: Serdyukov, P., et al. (eds.) ECIR 2013. LNCS, vol. 7814, pp. 816–819. Springer, Heidelberg (2013). https://doi.org/10.1007/978-3-642-36973-5_92

Automatic Text Classification for Label Imputation of Medical Diagnosis Notes Based on Random Forest

Bokai Yang[1,2], Guangzhe Dai[1], Yujie Yang[1], Darong Tang[1], Qi Li[1], Denan Lin[3], Jing Zheng[3(✉)], and Yunpeng Cai[1(✉)]

[1] Shenzhen Institutes of Advanced Technology,
Chinese Academy of Sciences, Shenzhen 518055, China
yp.cai@siat.ac.cn
[2] Northeastern University, Shenyang 110819, China
[3] Shenzhen Medical Information Center, Shenzhen 518000, China
cnzhengj@163.com

Abstract. Electronic medical records (EMRs) contain many information of patients, which are of great value for data mining for various clinical applications. However, information missing, including label missing, is pervasive in nature EMRs which would bring lots of obstacles for processing of the medical text contents. The aim of this study is to adopt automatic text classification technologies to recover missing medical text labels for EMRs and support downstream analyses. A combination of word-embedding technology and random forest classifiers are applied to identify multiple medical note labels including disease types and examination types, from short texts of medical imaging diagnosis notes. The results show that the average binary classification accuracies are 91%. Our research results indicate that using advanced NLP techniques for EMRs can reach high classification accuracies.

Keywords: Electronic medical record · Text information
Binary classification · Completion of missed information · Word2Vec
Random forest

1 Introduction

The electronic health record (EHR) is an evolving concept defined as a longitudinal collection of electronic health information about individual patients and populations [1]. An electronic medical record consists of both structured and unstructured data, where the unstructured data comprise free-style text such as the main symptoms, progress notes, and discharge summaries [2]. With the rapid increase in the number of patients, the number of electronic medical records has also become larger and larger, introducing more and more burdens to the efforts of medical text processing. Mistakes and information missing become common with the rapid increasing of data sizes, which might be caused by the following effects: (1) Manual errors: doctors may miss something when inputting electronic medical records, and this may cause the vocabulary gap and incomplete information. (2) Text parsing errors due to the complexities

S. Siuly et al. (Eds.): HIS 2018, LNCS 11148, pp. 87–97, 2018.
https://doi.org/10.1007/978-3-030-01078-2_8

of medical language characteristics, including (1) unrecognized medical jargons; (2) non-unified units or doses such as "mmHg" and "Kpa"; (3) numerous abbreviations such as "CT" and "MRI"; and (4) incomplete syntactic components of sentences [2]. (3) Information missing in data conversion due to heterogeneous database structures. EMR data missing key labels (i.e., annotation or subtitle information about record types, diagnosis types, disease codes, clinical instructions, etc.) would usually be excluded from clinical studies, which leads to a severe waste of resources. Imputing missing labels for these records would greatly improve the utilization of EMR systems.

The rapid growth of electronically available health related information, using natural language processing (NLP) and machine learning algorithms, have opened new opportunities for disease diagnosis and medical investigations [3, 4]. Information technology (IT) has become the principal vehicle that some believe will reduce medical error [1]. In particular, annotated corpora have become available to implement data-centric NLP algorithms and supervised machine learning techniques [5]. Computer models help doctors complete the diagnosis which are no given in electronic medical records [6]. Previously, people focused on the classification of medical images, such as breast lesions [7], lymph node recognition [8], esophageal cancer [9] and other people focused on text clustering [10, 11]. The power of machine learning and NLP techniques provides a possibility to automatically classify medical text records and impute the missing labels. However, until today there is still limited research attempts for this purpose.

The purpose of our study is to impute the diagnosis code and device type annotations in a large, practical medical text data set, which makes flexible matching and indexing of clinical cases for specified population studies possible in further steps. We use an in-house data set for the research tasks described in this paper. In this paper, we first constructed a data set of annotated Chinese electronic health records, and then presented a binary classification method based on Random Forest. The data set contains six kinds of entities, namely, the examination department, the device type, the Chinese name, the description, the result of the examination and the diagnosis. The method consists of two phases. In phase 1, the data set was pre-processed for representing the contents using word-embedding techniques. We segmented the data set into words and removed stop words at the same time. Then, these words are represented as vectors by word embedding. In phase 2, a binary classification method was built based on Random Forest. We treated the problem as a binary classification problem. And then we trained models for every pair of classes. Experimental results showed that our method can reach high classification accuracies. Further details are described in the following sections.

2   Materials and Methods

2.1   Material

The data used in this paper come from the Shenzhen regional medical information systems which incorporated medical records from various outpatients and hospitals. A total of 282740 notes describing medical imaging diagnosis results exist in the systems for registered hypertension patients, but only 15466 pieces of them are with complete diagnosis code and image type labels. That is to say, more than 90% of the diagnostic label information is missing. The 15466 notes with complete label information are used in our study for model training and validation, while the results would be applied to the rest of the records.

Table 1 illustrates an example of the text segment. According to the statistics, the data set includes 7855 males, 7006 females, and 545 unknowns. The proportion of men and women is basically 1:1. In addition, we also take a picture of the experimental data from the aspects of age distribution, distribution of disease categories, and distribution of device types. The specific distribution is shown in Table 2.

Table 1. An example of the text segment

Examination department	CCU
Device type	CT
Chinese name	冠状动脉CT平扫 (CT scan of coronary artery)
Description	冠状动脉平扫：右冠状动脉见钙化影。 冠状动脉增强：冠状动脉分布呈右优势型。(CT scan of coronary artery: Calcification in the right coronary artery. Enhancement of coronary artery: The distribution of coronary artery is right dominant)
Result	冠状动脉粥样硬化改变，右冠状动脉轻度狭窄。(Coronary artery atherosclerosis, mild coronary artery stenosis)
Diagnosis	冠心病 (coronary heart disease)

2.2 Methods

This section is divided into two broad subsections. In the first subsection, we provide detailed descriptions of the algorithms. In the second subsection, we discuss our automatic classification experiments in detail.

Word2Vec. In 2013, Google opened up a tool for word vector computing - Word2-Vec. Two particular models for learning word representations that can be efficiently trained on large amounts of text data are Continuous bag-of-words (CBOW) and Skip-gram models [12].

Continuous bag-of-words (CBOW). Unlike a language model that can only base its predictions on past words, as it is assessed based on its ability to predict each next word in the corpus, a model that only aims to produce accurate word-embedding is not subject to such restriction [13]. Therefore use both the n words before and after the target word w_t to predict it as shown in Fig. 1. This is known as a continuous bag of

Table 2. Data resource statistics

Age distribution	Number	Proportion
0–18	59	0.38%
19–30	1275	8.24%
31–50	5255	33.98%
51–70	5927	38.32%
Over 71	2692	17.41%
Unknown	258	1.67%
Distribution of disease types		
Coronary heart disease	3145	20.33%
Hypertension	2712	17.54%
Diabetes	2182	14.11%
Pulmonary tuberculosis	1620	10.47%
Abdominal pain	1157	7.48%
Others	4650	30.07%
Device types distribution		
US	7964	51.49%
CT	2165	14.00%
XR	1230	7.95%
GS	447	2.89%
MR	366	2.37%
Others	3294	21.30%

words (CBOW), owing to the fact that it uses continuous representations whose order is of no importance [14].

The purpose of CBOW is only marginally different than that of the language model one:

$$J_\theta = \frac{1}{T} \sum_{t=1}^{T} \log p(w_t | w_{t-n}, \ldots, w_{t-1}, w_{t+1}, \ldots, w_{t+n}) \tag{1}$$

Rather than feeding n previous words into the model, the model receives a window of n words around the target word w_t at each time step t.

Skip-gram. While CBOW can be seen as a precognitive language model, skip-gram turns the language model objective on its head: rather than using the surrounding words to predict the center word as with CBOW, skip-gram uses the center word to predict the surrounding words as can be seen in Fig. 2.

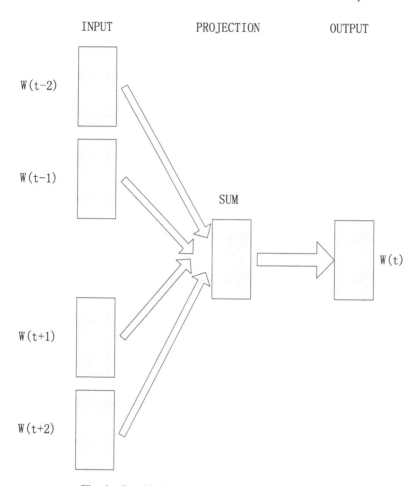

Fig. 1. Graphical representation of the CBOW model

The skip-gram objective thus sums the log probabilities of the surrounding n words to the left and to the right of the target word w_t to produce the following objective:

$$J_\theta = \frac{1}{T} \sum_{t=1}^{T} \sum_{-n \le j \le n, \ne 0} \log p(w_{t+j}|w_t) \qquad (2)$$

It was recently shown that the distributed representations of words capture surprisingly many linguistic regularities, and that there are many types of similarities among words that can be expressed as linear translations [12]. For example, vector operations "king" − "man" + "woman" results in a vector that is close to "queen".

Random Forest Random forests [15–17] refer to the establishment of a forest in a random manner, whereas forests contain multiple decision trees, and all decision trees are not related to each other. After training the random forest model, if there is a new

INPUT   PROJECTION   OUTPUT

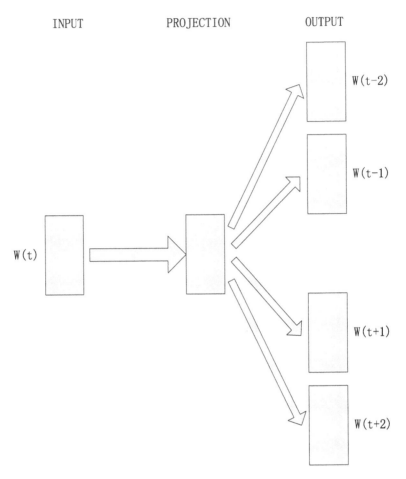

Fig. 2. Graphical representation of the Skip-gram model

data input, each decision tree in the random forest will classify it. Finally, which category is chosen to be more, it is categorized into that category.

Each tree is grown as follows [16]:

1. If the number of cases in the training set is N, sample N cases at random - but with replacement, from the original data. This sample will be the training set for growing the tree.
2. If there are M input variables, a number m ≪ M is specified such that at each node, m variables are selected at random out of the M and the best split on these m is used to split the node. The value of m is held constant during the forest growing.
3. Each tree is grown to the largest extent possible. There is no pruning.

In the original paper [15] on random forests, it was shown that the forest error rate depends on two things:

1. The correlation between any two trees in the forest. Increasing the correlation increases the forest error rate.
2. The strength of each individual tree in the forest. A tree with a low error rate is a strong classifier. Increasing the strength of the individual trees decreases the forest error rate.

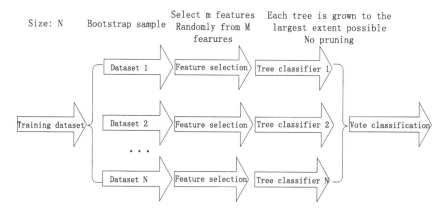

Fig. 3. The principle of random forest algorithm

Reducing m reduces both the correlation and the strength. Increasing it increases both. Somewhere in between is an "optimal" range of m - usually quite wide. Using the oob error rate a value of m in the range can quickly be found. This is the only adjustable parameter to which random forests is somewhat sensitive. Figure 3 shows the algorithm principle of a random forest.

TF-IDF as a Baseline Method. TF-IDF (term frequency–inverse document frequency) [18, 19] is a commonly used mathematical algorithm to assess the importance of a word for a particular piece of text segment in a data set. The more times a word appears in the text segment, the more important the word is. But the more times a word appears in the data set, the less important the word is.

The number of times a word appears in a text segment is referred to as word frequency. For the word ti, its importance can be expressed as formula 1:

$$\mathrm{tf}_{i,j} = \frac{n_{i,j}}{\sum_k n_{k,j}} \qquad (3)$$

In formula 1, $n_{i,j}$ is the times that ti appears in the data set d_j, The denominator represents the total number of words in d_j.

Inverse document frequency (IDF) represents the times a word appears in a data set. Specifically, IDF is equal to the number of text segments contained in a data set divided by the number of text segments that contain the word, and the obtained results are logarithmic. IDF can be expressed as formula 2:

$$idf_i = \log \frac{|D|}{|\{j : t_i \in d_j\}|} \tag{4}$$

$|D|$ represents the number of text segments contained in the data set. $|\{j : t_i \in d_j\}|$. represents the number of text segments contained the word.

At last, term frequency–inverse document frequency can be expressed as formula 3:

$$tfidf_{i,j} = tf_{i,j} * idf_i \tag{5}$$

Terms that are unique to specific text segments, get higher scores, while terms that are common throughout the corpus are assigned lower scores by this measure [20]. Therefore, TF-IDF can filter out common words such as "and" and "I" and leave important terms.

3 Experiment Setup

For the classification experiments, we divide the data set into two parts: 80% for training and 20% for evaluation [18]. These 80/20 splits are stratified, meaning that the proportions of positive cases and negative cases are the same as in the full data set. We now provide a detailed description of the text preprocessing approaches in Fig. 2.

Data Processing. First, the data is exported as a file in .csv format. We select positive cases and negative cases of non-CHD from the data set. Then we label the positive cases as 1 and the negative cases as 0. At the next, We segment the text [19] with the best Python Chinese word segmentation module - jieba. Some words are meaningless to the classification, such as punctuation and place name. So we remove the words [20] before the classification.

Set Up a Vector Space Model. We use word2vec to train the word embedding. The dimension of embedding is empirically set to 100 [20].We apply Word2Vec to map the texts to a matrix [21]. In this step, we use TF-IDF as the baseline algorithm to replace Word2Vec to map the texts to a matrix in the diagnosis group's experiment.

Set Up a Machine Learning Model and Test the Model. The above matrix is used as the feature. 80% of the data set is taken as the training set, and we apply a random forest to train the data. The remaining 20% data are used as the test set to test the trained data set (Fig. 4).

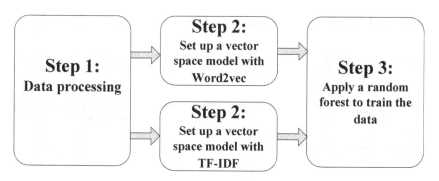

Fig. 4. A detailed description of the proposed text preprocessing approach and the baseline approach for comparison

4 Results

In this section, we provide details of the classification results of our experiments. We have done two groups of experiments, and each group contains 10 groups of binary experiments separately. The device type group's experimental results are shown in Table 3, and the diagnosis group's experimental results are shown in Table 4.

Table 3. F-score and accuracy of binary classification of diagnosis group

Distribution of disease types	Positive cases number	Positive cases F-score with Word2Vec/TF-IDF	Negative cases F-score with Word2Vec/TF-IDF	Test accuracy (%) with Word2Vec/TF-IDF)
US	4000	1.00/1.00	1.00/1.00	1.00/1.00
CT	2000	0.99/0.99	0.99/0.99	0.99/0.99
XR	1000	0.98/0.98	0.99/0.99	0.99/0.99
GS	400	1.00/1.00	1.00/1.00	1.00/1.00
MR	350	0.96/0.98	0.94/0.98	0.95/0.98

Table 4. F-score and accuracy of binary classification of device type group

Distribution of disease types	Positive cases number	Positive cases F-score with Word2Vec/TF-IDF	Negative cases F-score with Word2Vec/TF-IDF	Test accuracy (%) with Word2Vec/TF-IDF
Coronary heart disease	3000	0.86/0.84	0.85/0.84	0.86/0.84
Hypertension	2500	0.82/0.81	0.80/0.79	0.81/0.80
Diabetes	2000	0.97/0.94	0.96/0.94	0.96/0.94
Pulmonary tuberculosis	1500	1.00/1.00	0.99/1.00	1.00/1.00
Abdominal pain	1000	0.93/0/88	0.93/0.88	0.93/0.88

5 Conclusion and Discussion

In the device type group, our classifier get a 99% accuracy in average. In the diagnosis group, our classifier has the best classification effect for pulmonary tuberculosis, reaching a 100% accuracy rate. But the classifier is not good at classifying hypertension, and the accuracy rate is only 81%. Most classification accuracy rates are higher than 85%, and the average accuracy rate of our model is 91%, which is a relatively high accuracy rate. As you can see, the accuracy rate with TF-IDF is lower than the accuracy rate with Word2Vec in average.

In this paper we focused on the problem of automatic text classification for label imputation of the electronic medical records. We utilized NLP techniques to extract useful features from the data set and showed that the careful selection of features can reach high automatic classification accuracies. Our experiments showed that different labels can be distinguished on a large, real medical text data set. Therefore, we intend to use the established model to assist doctors in the completion of missed information in electronic medical records.

In the future, we want to explore what NLP and feature extraction techniques from text classification problems can be applied to text in the medical domain. From an NLP and more general medical informatics perspective, we will attempt to use deep learning to classify texts.

Acknowledgment. The work is supported in part by the NSFC funding 11471313, the Science and Technology Planning Project of Guangdong Province (2015B010129012) and the Shenzhen Basic Research Funding JCYJ20150630114942270.

References

1. Gunter, T.D., Terry, N.P.: The emergence of national electronic health record architectures in the United States and Australia: models, costs, and questions. J. Med. Internet Res. **7**(1), e3 (2005)
2. Dong, X., Qian, L., Guan, Y., et al.: A multiclass classification method based on deep learning for named entity recognition in electronic medical records. In: Scientific Data Summit, pp. 1–10. IEEE (2016)
3. Mujtaba, G., Shuib, L., Raj, R.G., et al.: Automatic ICD-10 multi-class classification of cause of death from plaintext autopsy reports through expert-driven feature selection. PLoS ONE **12**(2), e0170242 (2017)
4. Li, M., Fei, Z., Zeng, M., et al.: Automated ICD-9 coding via a deep learning approach. IEEE/ACM Trans. Comput. Biol. Bioinform. **PP**(99), 1 (2018)
5. Rajkomar, A., Oren, E., Chen, K., et al.: Scalable and accurate deep learning with electronic health records. npj Digit. Med. **1**(1), 18 (2018)
6. Rios, A., Kavuluru, R.: Convolutional neural networks for biomedical text classification: application in indexing biomedical articles. In: ACM BCB 2015, pp. 258–267 (2015)
7. Kooi, T., Litjens, G., Ginneken, B.V., et al.: Large scale deep learning for computer aided detection of mammographic lesions. Med. Image Anal. **35**, 303 (2016)

8. Roth, H.R., Lu, L., Seff, A., et al.: A new 2.5D representation for lymph node detection using random sets of deep convolutional neural network observations. Med. Image Comput. Comput. Assist. Interv. **17**(1), 520–527 (2014)

9. Ypsilantis, P.P., Siddique, M., Sohn, H.M., et al.: Predicting response to neoadjuvant chemotherapy with pet imaging using convolutional neural networks. PLoS ONE **10**(9), e0137036 (2015)

10. 胡浩, 李平, 陈凯琪. 基于汉字固有属性的中文字向量方法研究. 中文信息学报 **31**(3), 32–40 (2017)

11. Yu, D., Deng, L.: Feature representation learning in deep neural networks (2015)

12. Mikolov, T., Le, Q.V., Sutskever, I.: Exploiting similarities among languages for machine translation. Comput. Sci. (2013)

13. Mikolov, T., Chen, K., Corrado, G., et al.: Efficient estimation of word representations in vector space. Comput. Sci. (2013)

14. Goldberg, Y., Levy, O.: word2vec explained: deriving Mikolov et al.'s negative-sampling word-embedding method. Eprint Arxiv (2014)

15. Breiman, L.: Random forests. Mach. Learn. **45**(1), 5–32 (2001)

16. Cutler, A., Cutler, D.R., Stevens, J.R.: Random forests. Mach. Learn. **45**(1), 157–176 (2004)

17. Zimmerman, N., Presto, A.A., Kumar, S.P.N., et al.: A machine learning calibration model using random forests to improve sensor performance for lower-cost air quality monitoring. Atmos. Meas. Tech. **11**(1), 291–313 (2018)

18. Martineau, J., Finin, T.: Delta TFIDF: an improved feature space for sentiment analysis. In: International Conference on Weblogs and Social Media, ICWSM 2009, San Jose, California, USA. DBLP, May 2009

19. Soucy, P., Mineau, G.W.: Beyond TFIDF weighting for text categorization in the vector space model. In: International Joint Conference on Artificial Intelligence, pp. 1130–1135. Morgan Kaufmann Publishers Inc. (2005)

20. Sarker, A., Gonzalez, G.: Portable automatic text classification for adverse drug reaction detection via multi-corpus training. J. Biomed. Inform. **53**, 196–207 (2015)

21. Peng, K.H., Liou, L.H., Chang, C.S., et al.: Predicting personality traits of Chinese users based on Facebook wall posts. In: Wireless and Optical Communication Conference, pp. 9–14. IEEE (2015)

22. Saif, H., Fernandez, M., He, Y., et al.: On stopwords, filtering and data sparsity for sentiment analysis of twitter. In: The International Conference on Language Resources and Evaluation (2014)

23. Liu, Y., Ge, T., Mathews, K., et al.: Exploiting task-oriented resources to learn word embeddings for clinical abbreviation expansion. In: BioNLP 2015, pp. 92–97 (2015)

24. Rong, X.: word2vec Parameter Learning Explained. Comput. Sci. (2014)

An Automated Approach for Clinical Quantitative Information Extraction from Chinese Electronic Medical Records

Shanshan Liu[1], Xiaoyi Pan[1], Boyu Chen[1], Dongfa Gao[1(✉)], and Tianyong Hao[2(✉)]

[1] School of Informatics, Guangdong University of Foreign Studies, Guangzhou, China
shan63333@hotmail.com, Invy_pan@163.com,
JoeyChenby@163.com, gaodf@gdufs.edu.cn
[2] School of Computer Science, South China Normal University, Guangzhou, China
haoty@126.com

Abstract. Clinical quantitative information commonly exists in electronic medical records (EMRs) and is essential for recording patients' lab test or other characteristics in clinical notes. This study proposes an automated approach for extracting quantitative information from Chinese free-text EMR data including admission records, progress notes and ward-inspection records. The approach leverages pattern-learning combining with rule-based strategy to identify and extract clinical quantitative expressions. The experiments are based on 1,359 de-identified EMRs from the burn department of a domestic Grade-A Class-three hospital. The evaluation results present that our approach achieves a precision of 96.1%, a recall of 90.9%, and an F1-measure of 92.9%, demonstrating its effectiveness in clinical quantitative information extraction from EMR text.

Keywords: Clinical quantitative information · Electronic medical record
Natural language processing · Information extraction

1 Introduction

Quantitative information is analyzable textual expressions which are composed of entities related with numerical values and unit-based terms involving measurements [1]. As quantitative information describes entities and their associated numeric attributes, it plays an essential role for enhancing data analysis. In medical domain, it facilitates disease surveillance, dose study and advanced health research [2, 3]. According to statistics, quantitative information widely exists in medical text, for instance, more than 40% of free-text eligibility criteria contain numeric statements, as addressed in [4]. Whereas, most of them exist in free-text, leading to the bottleneck of utilizing those data directly in clinical research [5, 6].

Electronic medical record (EMR) is an electronically-stored record that collects the medical information of patients during treatment in hospital. Although it has a relatively structured writing specification, it includes free-text components including

© Springer Nature Switzerland AG 2018
S. Siuly et al. (Eds.): HIS 2018, LNCS 11148, pp. 98–109, 2018.
https://doi.org/10.1007/978-3-030-01078-2_9

admission records and discharge summaries that enable medical personnel to record particular situations of patients [7]. These unstructured components generate a lot of flexible expressions of natural language and increase the burden of the information extraction task. Another extraction challenge derives from the drawback of clinical text itself: (1) Omission of corresponding units, e.g., *"体温由39下降至37.5"* (Temperature dropped from 39 to 37.5), there is a unit *"摄氏度"* (Degrees Celsius) missing behind the digitals. (2) Misspelling problem, e.g., *"全身多处火焰烧伤70%%"* (Multiple body flame burns 70%%), the last "%" is redundant. (3) Irregularities expressions, e.g., *"创面剩余0.4%深二度创面"* (Wounds remaining 0.4% Deep II° wounds), the first *"创面"* (wounds) is redundant. Compared to EMR in English, certain particular challenges exist in information extraction tasks for Chinese unstructured EMR processing: (1) Chinese language has a particular linguistic property that words lack of distinct delimiter [8], thus word segmentation is needed toward word boundary identification. (2) A list of English medical repositories exist as comprehensive resource for named entity recognition, e.g., Unified Medical Language System (UMLS) [9], RxNorm [10]. However, there is no such relevant Chinese medical thesaurus [11]. (3) Due to the flexibility of Chinese EMR text representation, it is difficult to conduct syntax analysis for Chinese EMR text as English [12], even the syntax analysis has been proved to be effective in English EMR text extraction [13, 14]. With the massive use of EMRs, the scale of quantitative information of unstructured clinical data is rising rapidly. Therefore, it is imperative to extract quantitative information efficiently from clinical text.

In some existing studies [15–20], researchers extracted medication information which contained partial quantitative information such as dosage, frequency and duration from clinical free-text. Xu et al. [17] developed a system called MedEx to extract medical signature information including strength, route, and frequency from discharge summaries and the system achieved a high F-measure of 96%. Garvin et al. [20] used regular expressions combined with rules-based method to extract the left ventricular ejection fraction, an important index of cardiac insufficiency, from echocardiogram reports. Whereas, the above methods are only for the extraction of certain specific types of quantitative information. As to recording the physical condition of patients for disease surveillance or prevention, it still requires extracting complete numeric information of the medical records. Since quantitative information of the medical text is crucial for further analysis, some available methods were proposed to extract and format the numeric information into structured data. Voorham et al. [21] used a number-oriented approach to extract thirteen numeric medical measurements from electronic patient records. This approach compared every sentence in text with a list of numeric features by setting a four-word window. Nevertheless, there had no specific process for identifying unit and comparison operator related to the numeric. Bigeard et al. [22] used an automatic method by leveraging conditional random field (CRF) to identify numeric information and utilizing a rule-based method to associate entity and corresponding values. It reached precision of 96%, a recall of 78% and an F-measure of 86%. A drawback of this method was that it was burdensome to process a sentence including more than two numerical values and one of them missing necessary unit. Unlike the identification of the relations of entity pairs, there are no specific relations between entities and measures. Moreover, it is difficult to identify whether there is a relation or not between two extractions if the unit that related to numeric is missing. Thus, the traditional way using regular expressions combined with a rule-based strategy is time-consuming and it is hard to recognize the relations of entities and measures. Sohn et al. [23] analyzed the EMRs of Mayo Clinic and i2b2 challenge data, and found that the dominant patterns of the cross-institutional medical records were mutual. This finding denoted that the majority of medical information could be represented by certain patterns. According to some studies, pattern-based methods can improve the clinical information extraction, for instance, Aramaki et al. [24] utilized the patterns of discharge summaries to identify the relations of drug events and related effects. In term of Chinese clinical records, Xu et al. [25] proposed a hybrid method that used patterns to obtain the main lexica of Chinese medical terms and combined with SVM to extract time-event-description triples. The methods above are practicable but it is hard to comprehensively represent for the further information since they used lexica as the only feature of patterns. Thus, we proposed a new quantitative information extraction approach by using semantic as well as lexica for pattern-learning and integrating with rules-based method to overcome the quantitative information extraction barriers exhibited above.

To that end, we tagged key semantic roles of medical texts to generate patterns automatically, where the key semantic roles are used for the identification of comparison relations and further extraction. In addition, a matching algorithm was designed to calculate pattern matching score and processed sentences for enhancing extraction correctness. If the scores were lower than a certain threshold, a rule-based method was applied to jointly extract the quantitative information. We evaluated our approach by extracting three kinds of quantitative information from EMR free texts: physical examination index, dosage and diagnosis, which can present the physical condition of patients to a certain extent. The evaluation was based on 1,359 de-identified EMRs from the burn department of a domestic Grade-A Class-three hospital. The results with a high F1-measure of 92.2% demonstrated the outstanding performance of our approach.

2   The Approach

Considering that solely rule-based method may has the problem of lacking observation of context relations between entities and measures, we propose a hybrid approach that uses pattern-learning combined with rule-based method to extract quantitative information from clinical text. The extractions are represented as quad-tuples $NE = [E, C, N, U]$ and each element in the quad-tuple represents for entity (E), comparison operator (C), numeric (N), and related unit (U), respectively. The overall framework of our approach is shown in Fig. 1.

(1) **Text pre-processing**

Since a medical sentence was the basic unit to be processed in our approach, we used NLTK [26] - an open source NLP tool which contains sentence boundary detection module, and combined with some pre-defined rules to split text into sentences. The sentences with numeric features were identified by using a set of

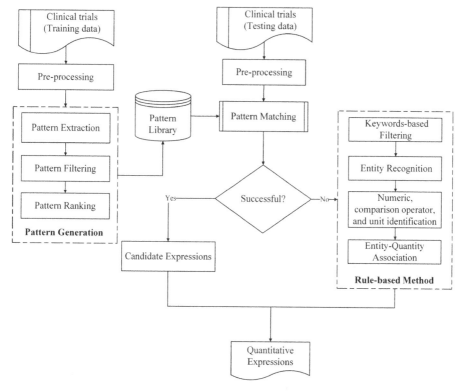

Fig. 1. The overall framework of our approach for clinical quantitative information extraction.

regular expressions, while others without these features were filtered out. Afterwards, we applied a widely used NLP tool - Jieba and combined it with a pre-defined medical dictionary for Chinese character segmentation. Eventually, every sentence was transformed into a word list W [w_1, w_2, w_3, w_4...w_n], where n represented for the length of the word list.

(2) **Pattern generation**

Initially, we used regular expressions and a pre-defined dictionary to tag three types of important information: entity, numeric, and unit as '$<E>$', '$<N>$', and '$<U>$' in the training data for further extraction. To a certain extent, whether or not there is a relation between entity and measure depends on the key semantic words that appear in a sentence. Hence, we tagged these words as corresponding labels as well. According to the description of the medical records, we divided these key semantic words into three categories: (1) words that represent for "larger than" relation between entity and measure tagged as '$<GR\_M>$'; (2) words that represent for "less than" relation tagged as '$<LW\_M>$'; (3) words that represent for "equal or approximately equal" relation tagged as '$<EQ\_M>$'. Besides, we found that the punctuation near to the extraction as a special sign is of vital importance. Thus, punctuations were tagged as '$<P>$'. The definitions of the semantic roles are described in Table 1.

Table 1. The definition and examples of the semantic roles used in our approach.

Semantic role	Tag	Definition	Example
Entity	*\<E>*	Medical mention, it includes drug name, inspection index and diagnosis	创面, 球蛋白
Numeric	*\<N>*	Various kinds of number types	37.5, 5.28 * 10^6
Unit	*\<U>*	The basis part for measurement	ml, °C
Equal	*\<EQ_M>*	A set of words that represents for equal or approximately equal relation	约, 达
Greater than	*\<GR_M>*	A kind of comparison operator that represents for "larger than" relation	超过, 以上
Lower than	*\<LW_M>*	A kind of comparison operator that represents for "less than" relation	低于, 以下
Punctuation	*\<P>*	Conventional signs that used to express a pause	。, :

For enabling each pattern to handle quantitative information corresponding to one medical mention better, it is necessary to determine the break point of the generated patterns. Specifically, if a pattern has more than one entity, the approach takes the first entity '$<E>$' that appears as the starting point of the determination and takes the next '$<N>$' label as intermediate sign and the next '$<E>$' label as final sign, splits the patterns into two sections from the final sign. For instance, in sentence *"双手电弧烧伤II°浅2% II°深1.7%."* (Electric arc burned of both hands Superficial II° 2% Deep II° 1.7%), the initial corresponding pattern is "[*双手, 电弧, 烧伤*, $<E>$, $<N>$, $<U>$, $<E>$, $<N>$, $<U>$, $<P>$]". After being treated with the rules above, the pattern is split into "[*双手, 电弧, 烧伤*, $<E>$, $<N>$, $<U>$]" and "[$<E>$, $<N>$, $<U>$, $<P>$]". Afterwards, we removed the stop words of the patterns by using a stop word list and got the preliminary patterns.

From the perspective of making the pattern more comprehensive, we optimized the preliminary patterns by the following operations. First of all, based on the consideration that the words which had a long distance to both entities and numerics had little influence on semantic relations, only the unlabeled words in front of the first tag unit to the last tag unit were remained. Secondly, the patterns derived from others or duplicated ones were removed, for example, the pattern "[*术后*, $<E>$, $<P>$, $<N>$, $<U>$, $<P>$]" is a derivative of pattern "[$<E>$, $<P>$, $<N>$, $<U>$]". Finally, we calculated both confidence and support scores of all the patterns by matching back to initial text. To ensure the reliability of the generated patterns, we empirically set the confidence metric as 0.6 and support metric as 4 to filter out the pattern which has the score lower than corresponding threshold, and sort the patterns by confidence in descending order. Eventually, 22 patterns were generated and added to the pattern library. Some examples of the final pattern library are shown in Table 2.

Table 2. Some pattern examples with support and confidence scores.

Patterns	Support	Confidence
面积 <N> <U> <E> <P>	6	1.0
烫伤 <N> <U> <E> <P>	38	1.0
<E> <N> <U> <GR_M> <P>	6	1.0
覆盖 <N> <U> <E> <P>	4	1.0
<E> <P> <N> - <N> <U> <P>	20	1.0
覆盖面积 <N> <U> <E> <P>	4	1.0
<E> 最高 <EQ_M> <N> <U> <P>	5	1.0
检查 <P> <E> <EQ_M> <N> <U>	8	1.0
<E> 最高 <N> <U> <P>	26	1.0
<E> <N> - <N> <U> <P>	86	0.942
<E> <N> <U>	2542	0.937
<E> <EQ_M> <N> <U> <P>	94	0.936
<EQ_M> <N> <U> <E> <P>	24	0.917
<E> <EQ_M> <N> - <N> <U> <P>	10	0.9
烧伤 <N> <U> <E>	58	0.897
<E> <P> <N> <U>	199	0.658

(3) **Pattern matching**

Different from the traditional matching algorithm which match the sentence from the first place, we used keyword as the start point to match the wordlist from both left and right directions. As numeric is crucial for quantitative information extraction, we picked '<N>' as the matching keyword. Regarding wordlist as target string and pattern as pattern string, the pattern matching calculation is shown in Eqs. 1 to 4.

$$PScore(k, j) = \sum \sum_{left} f(PAT_{ki}, WL_j) + \sum \sum_{right} f(PAT_{ki}, WL_j) \quad (1)$$

$$f(\alpha, \beta) = \begin{cases} 1, \alpha \in M^*, Map(\beta) \notin N^* \wedge \beta \notin \Phi \\ q(\alpha, Map(\beta)), \; else \end{cases} \quad (2)$$

$$q(\gamma, \delta) = \begin{cases} 0, \gamma = \delta \\ 1, \; else \end{cases} \quad (3)$$

$$PAssess(k) = \begin{cases} PAT_k \Rightarrow Matched \; pattern, \; \exists PScore(k,j) = Len(PAT_k) \\ PAT_k \nRightarrow Matched \; pattern, \; \nexists PScore(k,j) = Len(PAT_k) \end{cases} \quad (4)$$

In the above equations, *PScore* denotes the matching score of current pattern list after comparing the left and right direction of touch point of the target string with pattern string. PAT_{ki} denotes the element in the location i of pattern k. WL_j denotes the element in the location j of target string. $f(\alpha, \beta)$ calculates the score after comparison. M^* denotes the assemblage of role labels $<E>$ and $<U>$. N^* denotes the assemblage of the rest role labels. $Map(\beta)$ maps word into corresponding semantic role label ($<EQ\_M>$, $<GR\_M>$, $<LW\_M>$, or $<p>$) on the premise that it is key semantic word or else keep it as the same. $q(\gamma, \delta)$ judges the identical of γ (the corresponding word in pattern k) and δ (the corresponding word in target string). $PAssess$ denotes the final match result of the target string and pattern k. $Len(PAT_k)$ denotes the length of the pattern k.

To describe the process, a specific work flow is presented in Fig. 2, where m2 to m8 represent different words. The approach automatically matched the left and right directions of the touch point (m4) of the target string with the pattern string. If the calculated score equals to the length of pattern string, a pattern is matched. Otherwise, the touch point will move to next $<N>$ tag and assess as above. This process is repeated until all the $<N>$ tags of the target string being went through. After extracting the information by pattern matching, a list of rules are applied to further process numeric information and represent it as quad-tuples.

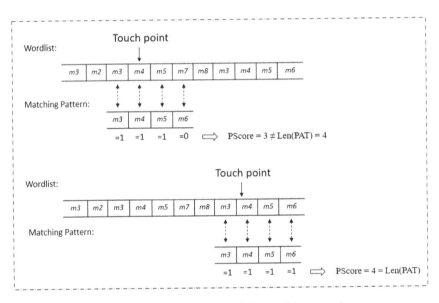

Fig. 2. The specific work flow of the matching procedure.

(4) **Rule-based method**

In case there is no pattern matched, a rule-based method will be applied to process the sentence which has the semantic tag '$<EQ\_M>$', '$<GR\_M>$' or '$<LW\_M>$'. The specific procedure can be conclude into 4 steps: (1) Applying regular expressions to recognize numerics in the sentence, e.g., $(\backslash d+)(\backslash.\backslash d+|)(|\backslash*(|)(\backslash d+)$ $(\backslash\backslash d+|)(\backslash\wedge)(\backslash d+)$ to identify scientific notation like 5.7 * 10^2 and $(\backslash d+)(\backslash.\backslash d+|)$ $(\backslash d+|)(|)(-)(|)(\backslash d+)(\backslash.\backslash d+|)(\backslash d+|)$ to identify a kind of number combination like '76–90'. (2) A domain knowledge including formal representations and common expressions is built to identify entities and units since they often have various kinds of representations, e.g., the unit of temperature can be *'°C'*, *'°'* or *'摄氏度'* (Degrees Celsius). (3) For the appearance of comparison operators are routine, we designed rules for extracting the compared relation of the measures. (4) Recognizing the associations between entities and measures. According to clinical record writing conventions, we defined rules that associated the nearest value pair preferentially, e.g., *M1-E1-E2-M2* to represent the sequence of the appearance of measures and entities, the association come out to be (*E1*, *M1*) and (*E2*, *M2*). To this end, numeric information quad-tuples were formed.

3   The Experiments and Results

3.1   Datasets

Our data came from the burn department of a domestic Grade-A Class-three hospital, containing a total of 1,359 de-identified EMRs (7,825 sentences in total). Those EMRs were divided into three types: admission records, progress notes and ward-inspection records. The extractions can be concluded into three categories: (1) physical examination index; (2) dosage; and (3) diagnosis. 56% of the clinical narratives (759 EMRs) were chosen as training data, and the rest 44% (600 EMRs) as testing data randomly. Three annotators including two clinical researchers and one data engineer manually annotated the testing dataset independently. For instance, *"右大腿热接触伤1%三度"* (1% three degrees of hot contact injury in the right thigh) was annotated as *"右大腿热接触伤<N>1</N><U>%</U><E>三度</E>"*. After the annotation, about 25% of total annotations are inconsistent. We solved all the inconsistency by consulting a senior clinician and formed a gold standard (1,950 quantitative expressions).

We utilized precision, recall, and F1-measure as three indicators to evaluate the performance [27]. Precision is defined as the ratio of correct expressions to all extracted expressions as True Positive/(True Positive + False Positive), where True Positive denotes the number of correct expressions while False Positive denotes the number of incorrect expressions among extracted ones. Recall is defined as the ratio of correct expressions to gold stand expressions as True Positive/(True Positive + False Negative), where False Negative denotes for the number of correct expressions failed to be extracted. F1-measure is defined as 2 * Precision * Recall/(Precision + Recall).

3.2   The Results

Our approach ran on the testing dataset with EMRs increasing from 50 to 600 while quantitative expressions rising from 111 to 1,950. Then, the precision, recall, and F1-measure of the different EMR data were calculated. As shown in Fig. 3, since the testing datasets reflected the increasing number of medical free-text, the F1-measure values had 1.3% variance after the 100 EMRs dataset. Based on the largest dataset containing 600 EMRs, the approach reached a precision of 0.961, a recall of 0.900, and an

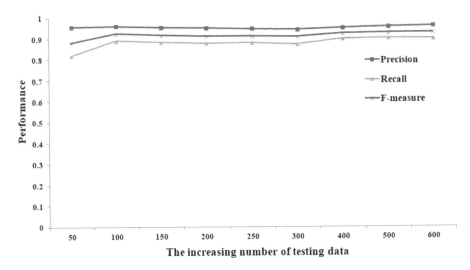

Fig. 3. The performance of our approach with increasing number of testing data.

F1-measure of 0.929. The results illustrated that our approach achieved stable performance on all evaluation metrics.

To demonstrate the effectiveness of integrating pattern-learning and rule-based method, we compared the performance of our approach with the rule-based only method and the pattern-based only method on the whole testing dataset. As shown in Table 3, the results of the rule-based only method got an F1-measure of 88.0% and a high recall of 90.9%, but a relatively mediocre precision of 85.2%. On the contrary, the pattern-based only method achieved an F1-measure of 90.8%, the best precision of 96.5%, but the lowest recall of 85.7%. Thus, our hybrid approach obtained a superior performance, evidencing its effectiveness.

Table 3. Comparison of performances of different approches.

Approach	Precision (%)	Recall (%)	F1-measure (%)
Rules	0.852	0.909	0.880
Pattern	0.965	0.857	0.908
Our method (Pattern + Rules)	0.961	0.900	0.929

4   Discussions

Under the consideration that few studies concentrated on quantitative information extraction from Chinese EMRs, it could be hard to carry out a comprehensive analysis for comparison with other researches. Aiming to further understand the performance of our method, we analyzed the experiment results. The rule-based only method has a relatively low precision while the pattern-based only method has a slightly weaker recall. The main cause for the phenomenon is that rule-based method used regular expression which has the limitation of processing sentences with complex relation of the entities and measures. Thus, it might generate the expression which has the wrong association of the entity and measure and reduced the precision as a result, e.g., *"2. 浅 II ° 烧伤：局部红肿明显"* (2. Superficial II ° burn: local swelling is evident), it mistakenly regarded the order number "2" as the quantity of the entity *"浅 II ° 烧伤"* (Superficial II ° burn). With respect to the pattern-based only method, numeric information will be extracted only when the sentence could match with the pattern of pattern library. Nevertheless, if the structure of the sentence has appearances less than the threshold we defined, it cannot be extracted. Consequently, it guaranteed the high accuracy but with low recall as price. Therefore, in this study we proposed a hybrid approach that pattern matching as dominative procedure combined with rule-based method to extract the quantitative information and it achieved an obvious improvement in the outcome.

We further analyzed the extraction errors of our hybrid approach and identified the mainly errors types are as follows. (1) The selection of boundary symbols. Since most of the entities and their related measures appeared in the sentences that used comma as boundary symbol, we defined comma as one of the boundary symbols, thus some entities and corresponding quantities that contained in different sentences could not be extracted. For example, the text *"血氧饱和度平静时100%，哭闹时达98%"* (Oxygen saturation is 100% when calming, and 98% when crying) had two quantities. Since *"98%"* is in another sentence, only the first measure *"100%"* was identified and associated with *"血氧饱和度"* (Oxygen saturation). (2) The recognition of named entity. We reviewed the error statements and found that most of the errors belong to diagnosis. The descriptions of diagnosis had various kinds of representations, e.g., some used narrative way to describe the diagnosis instead of specific nouns. For example, the text *"右上下肢热液烫伤13%"* (Right upper and lower limb hydrothermal burns 13%) had no named entity to associate with *"13%"*, but it actually presented that the extent of burn was 13%. As medical mentions were complicated and one entity might contain another entity name inside, e.g., *"葡萄糖6—磷酸脱氢酶"* (Glucose 6-phosphate dehydrogenase), our approach mistakenly identified '6' as the quantity of the entity *"葡萄糖"* (Glucose).

5 Summary

Targeting at extracting quantitative information from free-text EMRs, this research proposed an automated approach for high accurate quantitative information extraction from EMRs. Our approach generates structural patterns automatically and utilizes a rule-based method jointly for extracting and normalizing quantitative expressions from manually-annotated free text EMRs. Experiments on the real EMRs data from the burn department of a domestic Grade-A Class-three hospital show that our proposed approach outperforms the baseline methods, demonstrating the effectiveness of the approach.

Acknowledgements. This work was supported by National Natural Science Foundation of China (No. 61772146), Innovative School Project in Higher Education of Guangdong Province (No. YQ2015062), and Guangzhou Science Technology and Innovation Commission (No. 201803010063).

References

1. Hao, T., Wei, Y., Qiang, J., Wang, H., Lee, K.: The representation and extraction of quantitative information. In: ISO-ACL Workshop at the 12th International Conference on Computational Semantics (IWCS 2017), pp. 74–83 (2017)
2. Evans, D.A., Brownlow, N.D., Hersh, W.R., Campbell, E.M.: Automating concept identification in the electronic medical record: an experiment in extracting dosage information. In: A Conference of the American Medical Informatics Association, pp. 388–392 (1996)
3. Hassanpour, S., Langlotz, C.P.: Information extraction from multi-institutional radiology reports. Artif. Intell. Med. **66**, 29–39 (2016)
4. Hao, T., Liu, H., Weng, C.: Valx: a system for extracting and structuring numeric lab test comparison statements from text. Methods Inf. Med. **55**(3), 266–275 (2016)
5. Wang, Y., Wang, L., Rastegarmojarad, M., et al.: Clinical information extraction applications: a literature review. J. Biomed. Inform. **77**, 34–49 (2017)
6. Mykowiecka, A., Marciniak, A.: Rule-based information extraction from patients' clinical data. J. Biomed. Inform. **42**(5), 923–936 (2009)
7. Mcdonald, C.J.: The barriers to electronic medical record systems and how to overcome them. J. Am. Med. Inform. Assoc. JAMIA **4**(3), 213 (1997)
8. Wong, K.F., Li, W., Xu, R., Zhang, Z.S.: Introduction to Chinese natural language processing. Synth. Lect. Hum. Lang. Technol. **2**(1), 1–148 (2009)
9. Bodenreider, O.: The unified medical language system (UMLS): integrating biomedical terminology. Nucl. Acids Res. **32**(Suppl_1), 267–270 (2004)
10. Liu, S., Ma, W., Moore, R., Ganesan, V., Nelson, S.: RxNorm: prescription for electronic drug information exchange. IT Prof. **7**(5), 17–23 (2005)
11. Xu, Y., Wang, Y., Sun, J.T., Zhang, J., Tsujii, J., Chang, E.: Building large collections of Chinese and English medical terms from semi-structured and encyclopedia websites. PLoS ONE **8**(7), e67526 (2013)
12. Jiang, Z., Zhao, F., Guan, Y.: Developing a linguistically annotated corpus of Chinese electronic medical record. In: IEEE International Conference on Bioinformatics and Biomedicine, pp. 307–310. IEEE (2014)
13. de Bruijn, B., Cherry, C., Kiritchenko, S., Martin, J., Zhu, X.: Machine-learned solutions for three stages of clinical information extraction: the state of the art at i2b2 2010. J. Am. Med. Inform. Assoc. **18**(5), 557–562 (2011)
14. Fan, J.W., et al.: Syntactic parsing of clinical text: guideline and corpus development with handling ill-formed sentences. J. Am. Med. Inform. Assoc. **20**(6), 1168–1177 (2013)
15. Uzuner, Ö., Solti, I., Cadag, E.: Extracting medication information from clinical text. J. Am. Med. Inform. Assoc. JAMIA **17**(5), 514 (2010)
16. Gold, S., Elhadad, N., Zhu, X., Cimino, J.J., Hripcsak, G.: Extracting structured medication event information from discharge summaries. In: AMIA Annual Symposium Proceedings/AMIA Symposium, vol. 2008, pp. 237–241 (2008)

17. Xu, H., Stenner, S.P., Doan, S., Johnson, K., Waitman, L., Denny, J.: MedEx: a medication information extraction system for clinical narratives. J. Am. Med. Inform. Assoc. **17**(1), 19–24 (2010)
18. Patrick, J., Li, M.: High accuracy information extraction of medication information from clinical notes: 2009 i2b2 medication extraction challenge. J. Am. Med. Inform. Assoc. **17**(5), 524–527 (2010)
19. Xu, H., Doan, S., Birdwell, K.A., et al.: An automated approach to calculating the daily dose of tacrolimus in electronic health records. In: Amia Joint Summits on Translational Science Proceedings Amia Summit on Translational Science, vol. 2010, p. 71 (2010)
20. Garvin, J.H., et al.: Automated extraction of ejection fraction for quality measurement using regular expressions in Unstructured Information Management Architecture (UIMA) for heart failure. J. Am. Med. Inform. Assoc. **19**(5), 859–866 (2012)
21. Voorham, J., Denig, P.: Computerized extraction of information on the quality of diabetes care from free text in electronic patient records of general practitioners. J. Am. Med. Inform. Assoc. **14**(3), 349–354 (2007)
22. Bigeard, E., Jouhet, V., Mougin, F., Thiessard, F., Grabar, N.: Automatic extraction of numerical values from unstructured data in EHRs. Stud. Health Technol. Inform. **210**, 50–54 (2015)
23. Sohn, S., et al.: Analysis of cross-institutional medication description patterns in clinical narratives. Biomed. Inform. Insights **6**(Suppl 1), 7–16 (2013)
24. Eiji, A., et al.: Extraction of adverse drug effects from clinical records. Stud. Health Technol. Inform. **160**(Pt 1), 739 (2010)
25. Xu, D., et al.: Data-driven information extraction from Chinese electronic medical records. PLoS ONE **10**(8), e0136270 (2015)
26. Loper, E., Bird, S.: NLTK: the natural language toolkit. In: Proceedings of the ACL-02 Workshop on Effective Tools and Methodologies for Teaching Natural Language Processing and Computational Linguistics, vol. 1, pp. 63–70. Association for Computational Linguistics (2002)
27. Manning, C.D., Raghavan, P., Schütze, H.: Introduction to Information Retrieval. Cambridge University Press, Cambridge (2009)

A New Way of Channel Selection in the Motor Imagery Classification for BCI Applications

Md. A. Mannan Joadder[1], Siuly Siuly[2(✉)], and Enamul Kabir[3]

[1] Department of Electrical and Electronics Engineering,
United International University, Dhaka, Bangladesh
joaddermannan@gmail.com, sojol91@yahoo.com
[2] Center for Applied Informatics, College of Engineering and Science,
Victoria University, Melbourne, Australia
siuly.siuly@vu.edu.au
[3] Faculty of Health, Engineering and Sciences,
University of Southern Queensland, Toowoomba, QLD 4350, Australia
Enamul.Kabir@usq.edu.au

Abstract. Nowadays, motor imagery classification in electroencephalography (EEG) based brain computer interface (BCI) systems is a very important research topic in the study of brain science. As EEG contains multi-channel EEG recordings with huge amount of data, it is sometimes very challenging to extract more representative information from original EEG data for efficient classification of motor imagery (MI) tasks. Thus, it is necessary to diminish the redundant information from the original EEG signal selecting appropriate channels and also to reduce computational cost. Addressing this problem, we intend to develop a methodology based on channel selection for classification of MI tasks in the BCI applications. In this study, we introduce a new way of channel selection considering anatomical and functional structural of the human brain and also investigate its impact in the classification performance. In this proposed method, at first we select the channels from motor cortex area, and then decompose EEG signals using wavelet energy function into several bands of real and imaginary coefficients. The relevant band's coefficient energy has been used as feature vector in this research. After that, the extracted features are tested by three popular machine learning method: Linear Discriminant Analysis (LDA), Support Vector Machine (SVM) and K-Nearest Neighbour (KNN). The method is evaluated on a benchmark dataset IVa (BCI competition III) and the results demonstrate classification improvement with less computational cost over the existing methods.

Keywords: Electroencephalogram (EEG)
Independent Component Analysis (ICA) · Wavelet energy · SVM classifier

1 Introduction

Brain Computer Interface (BCI) is a system by which people can control electronic device such as a computer cursor, a robotic arm or even cell phone using their thoughts. The ultimate goal of BCI research is to assist the people who suffer from severe motor

© Springer Nature Switzerland AG 2018
S. Siuly et al. (Eds.): HIS 2018, LNCS 11148, pp. 110–119, 2018.
https://doi.org/10.1007/978-3-030-01078-2_10

disabilities. The BCI system basically creates an alternate communication channel by which one can easily communicate with the external world [23]. In BCI system, the commands that send to the external world do not pass through the brain's regular output paths of nerves and muscles [1, 26]. The system is capable of reading and translating the patient's intend to the physical commands which can control the external devices [24, 25].

This study focuses on motor imagery (MI) based BCI using EEG. The motor imagery based BCI is capable of translating the subject's movement intention to controls the external devices [2, 26]. According to the previous studies in MI based BCI, the movement imagination and actual movement produce the similar brain pattern over the sensorimotor cortex [2, 3]. These are known as Event Related Synchronization (ERS) and Event Related Desynchronization (ERD). These cause increase and decrease of EEG signal power in certain frequency bands. In the motor cortex regions these event related potentials occur. To attain a good accuracy in the classification of MI tasks, electrodes should place in the motor cortex region. From the previous research it is clear that only two electrodes, C3 and C4, which are located in the left and right motor cortex respectively, are capable to attain the maximum classification accuracy for MI tasks [4]. However, the large number of electrodes poses some issue like higher computational cost, additional artifacts and redundant information in the signal [5]. Hence it is very important to choose the optimal number of channels to address these problems. Lim et al. [6] used single electrode and find the best result for KNN classifier which is 72%. Shan et al. [7] reported the MI tasks classification results for different number of channels. According to his experiment it is clear that when he increases the electrode number from 16 to 59 the classification accuracy of testing data decreases from 81.3% to 68.9%. Oh et al. [8] reported the classification accuracy of 74.7% and 71.6% for SIFT and Hjorth parameter feature respectively while using three EEG electrodes. Resalat et al. [9] applied three electrodes for the classification of MI tasks for different features. He reported the maximum classification accuracy for the features Auto-Regressive (AR), Mean Absolute Value (MAV), and Band Power (BP) which is 75%. Yang et al. [10] employed six EEG electrodes for the classification of left hand, right hand and right foot motor imagery task classification. He reported the classification accuracy of 70.3% using WPBBD method.

The ultimate goal of this study is to decrease the number of EEG electrodes at the same time improve the classification accuracy and also reduce the computational cost. In our experiment we have proposed an efficient BCI method which can decrease the computational cost at the same time improve the classification accuracy. According to our knowledge no previous work has applied this method. We have proposed to use three channels with Independent Component Analysis (ICA) and SVM as the classifier. In our proposed method we have used the wavelet based sub-band energy as the feature vector. Most of the previous studies have shown that the classification accuracy increases by increasing the number of electrodes [11]. In contrast our proposed method can increase the classification accuracy by decreasing the number of electrodes.

2   Methodology

2.1   Problem Statement

To develop a BCI analysis tool which is capable of detect MI tasks, we have select channel wisely, filter the EEG signals for specific frequency band, remove the artifacts from signal using spatial filter, extract feature for better detection of MI tasks, use an appropriate classification method to discriminate the MI tasks, and then evaluate how efficient the analysis method is.

Given a set of labelled EEG signals from 2 classes, we want to be able to detect a new test set of signal into a specific class based on the pattern of the available training signals.

2.2   Channel Selection

Brain activities record as multichannel time series in EEG from different electrodes placed on the scalp of a person. The information that provided by the different electrodes does not contain the similar information [13]. In this study, we are interested to examine the performance of the different electrodes which are more related to the MI tasks. For this purpose we compare the classification accuracies of EEG electrodes from motor cortex area with the performance of the electrodes from other areas, as we know motor cortex area is very much related with voluntary muscle movements [14].

The purpose of this study is to compare the performance of our proposed method with all the other electrodes. That is why we divide our whole experiment into three cases.

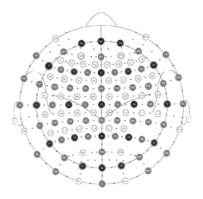

Fig. 1. Case-I (118 electrodes)

Figure 1 shows the case-I where we consider 118 channels from the whole scalp. This channel set up was provided by the data set. Several researchers have used this channel set up for the classification of MI tasks [15].

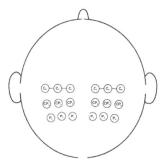

Fig. 2. Case-II (18 electrodes)

Figure 2 shows the set up for case-II which consists of 18 channels from motor cortex area. We manually selected these 18 EEG electrodes based on the placement of international 10/20 system. The channels included in this set up are: C5, C3, C1, C2, C4, C6, CP5, CP3, CP1, CP2, CP4, CP6, P5, P3, P1, P2, P4 and P6. Many researchers have considered these electrodes for MI tasks classification [14].

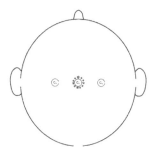

Fig. 3. Case-III (3 electrodes)

Figure 3 represents the set up for case-III. In this case, we considered only three channels named C3, C4 and Cz. According to our knowledge these channels contain more relevant information for the classification of MI tasks [16].

Finally we compared the classification accuracy of these three set of channels.

2.3 Independent Component Analysis (ICA)

It is known that EEG signals are noisy because of the spatial overlapping of activities which arises from the different brain regions. For addressing this problem spatial filter is required. Apart from that EEG signal is contaminated with the artifacts which produces from various source like muscle movement, eye blink etc. Independent Component Analysis (ICA) is capable of extracting the relevant information which is buried with the noisy signal. This is a statistical method which was first developed to solve the 'Cocktail Party Problem' [17]. Recent studies are using this method in BCI applications [18]. ICA can enhance the signal-to-noise ratio (SNR). Here, the description and calculation principal of ICA is given [19].

The observed signal $x(t)$ is the linear mixture of a statistically independent source signal $s(t)$

$$x(t) = As(t) \qquad (1)$$

where A is the mixing matrix. The columns of matrix A represent a spatial description for each of the Independent Components in s $s(t)$. This can be solved by estimating a suitable de-mixing matrix $W = A^{-1}$ which estimates the source waveforms by

$$s(t) = Wx(t) \qquad (2)$$

2.4   Feature Extraction

Wavelet Based Sub-Band Energy: The wavelet decomposition splits the original EEG signal into two subspaces. Complementary to each other, one subspace contains the low-frequency information of the original signal and the other one contains the high-frequency information of the original signal [20]. Figure 4 illustrates the wavelet decomposition system.

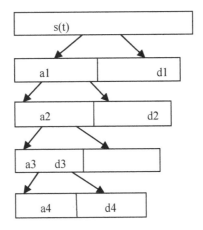

Fig. 4. Wavelet Decomposition Upto Level 4

After the wavelet decomposition the wavelet based sub band energy features are extracted. Here we use the wavelet function 'db4' for wavelet decomposition and the signals are decomposed up to level 4 as shown in Fig. 1. From each of the sub band energy features have been calculated.

2.5   Classification and Cross Validation

In this study three popular classifiers are used for comparing the performance of the proposed method. Here we included Linear Discriminant Analysis (LDA) [30, 32, 33], Support Vector Machine (SVM) [27–29, 31] and K-Nearest Neighbour (KNN) [28, 31]. A 10 × 10 fold cross validation is used to estimate the classification accuracy.

3   Experiments and Results

3.1   Experiment Setup

Band pass filtering and window size selection are necessary as we know only alpha and beta band are more related to MI tasks. In our study we select the window of size 3 s, which starts 0.5 s after the visual cue. To obtain higher classification performance the EEG signals are band pass filtered from 8–30 Hz using a Butterworth filter of order 5 [21]. Then the signals are pre-processed using ICA spatial filter as we discussed in Sect. 2. Then we extract wavelet based sub band energy feature for each of the channel. Finally, three types of classifier are used to solve the classification problem. We applied the same setup for all the three cases (case-I: consider 118 channels, case-II: manually select 18 channels, case-III: only three channels are selected). We used all three classifier for each of the case to compare the performance of the classifiers. That is why we reported three results for each of the case. The 10 × 10 fold cross validation procedure is used to evaluate the performance of the channels on the basis of classification accuracy.

3.2   Data Description

The experiment is performed based on BCI Competition III dataset IVa [12]. The data was recorded from five healthy subjects while performing right hand and right foot MI tasks. The signals were recorded using 118 channels (Extended 10/20) system. During the recording, subjects sat on comfortable chairs with arms resting on armrests. The sampling rate of the provided data was 1 kHz, but for our study we down sampled to 100 Hz. There are 280 trails of each subject among them 140 trial for each class. Each trial contains a recording of 3.5 s of any one of the MI tasks.

The classification results of five subjects are listed in Table 1. From the above table it is observed that the classification accuracy increases by decreasing the number of channels wisely. Considering SVM classifier the average result for case-I, case-II and case-III are 50.4%, 54.7% and 76% respectively. So from the average result of three cases we can see that the classification accuracy is lower in case-I, a little bit higher in case-II and the maximum in case-III. The other two classifiers also follow the same pattern. So it clear that maximum classification accuracy is obtained for case-III.

Among all the subjects it is observed that "al" performs best for case-III while using SVM classifier which is 91%. The same subject shows the classification accuracy of 51.7% for both the cases (case-I and case-II) using the classifier SVM. For subject "aa" the classification accuracy for three cases (case-I, case-II and case-III) are 53.2%, 59.6% and 61.4% respectively for using LDA classifier. The classification accuracy of

Table 1. For whole dataset (118 channels): overall classification performance (%) on dataset Iva

Case	Methods	aa	al	av	aw	ay	Mean	SD
I	SVM	53.5	51.7	48.9	44.6	53.5	50.4	3.7
	LDA	53.2	49.6	45.7	45.7	52.1	49.2	3.5
	KNN	53.2	55.0	45.7	**44.2**	47.5	49.1	4.7
II	SVM	62.1	51.7	49.6	63.5	46.7	54.7	7.5
	LDA	59.6	54.6	51.0	62.8	50.0	55.6	5.5
	KNN	55.7	56.7	47.1	51.4	48.9	51.9	4.1
III	SVM	59.2	**91.0**	58.5	83.5	87.8	**76.0**	15.8
	LDA	61.4	88.9	58.2	82.8	86.7	75.6	14.6
	KNN	55.3	80.7	56.7	76.7	80.3	69.9	12.8

aa = Subject1; al = Subject2; av = Subject3; aw = Subject4;
ay = Subject5; SD = Standard Deviation.
bold answers symbolizes the subject wise lowest, highest and
mean maximum result.

subject "av" for three cases (case-I, case-II and case-III) are 45.7%, 51.0% and 58.2% respectively when using the LDA classifier. Subject "aw" and "ay" also shows the same pattern for the three cases. It can be concluded that our proposed method can improve the classification accuracy significantly for all the subjects.

If we compare the performance of the classifiers from the average result it is clear that SVM classifier is the best performer for all the cases except case-II. The LDA classifier performs best in this specific case.

Therefore, it can be said that SVM classifier using three manually selected channels is the best combination for MI tasks classification.

Figure 5 compares the time consumption of three cases (case-I, case-II and case-III). From the above figure it is seen that the time consumption is maximum for the case-I. SVM classifier consumes the highest time for case-I which is 19.21 min. The same classifier spends 4.23 and 1.68 min for case-II and case-III respectively. The computational cost of LDA classifier is higher for case-I which is 17.91 min. The cost for other two cases is 4.06 and 1.59 min respectively. The KNN classifier shows the same pattern as like as the other classifiers mentioned earlier.

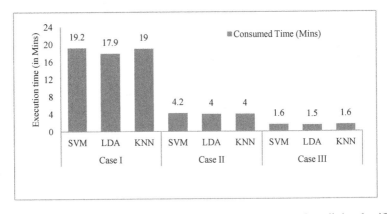

Fig. 5. Comparative study of time consumption for three cases using all the classifiers

From the above analysis it is clear that we can reduce the computational latency significantly by choosing the number of electrodes wisely.

4 Comparative Study

In this section we intend to show comparative study of our proposed method with existing method. Figure 6 shows the comparative results of different methods used by the researchers and our proposed method. Baziyad et al. [22] applied SVM for three class MI tasks classification and reported an average accuracy of 75%.

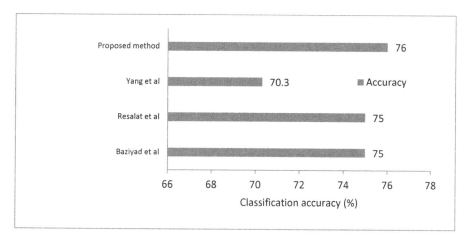

Fig. 6. Comparative studies of existing methods with our proposed method

Oh et al. [8] used three EEG channels for MI tasks classification and reported the result 74.7% and 71.6% for SIFT and Hjorth parameter feature respectively. The average classification accuracy for his proposed method was 79.1%. Resalat et al. [9] used C3, C4 and Cz electrodes in his experiment for different feature and reported the higher accuracy is 75%. Yang et al. [10] examined a method based on wavelet packet best basis decomposition. In his study he used six channels from primary sensorimotor cortex area. He reported the classification accuracy of 70.3%. Our proposed method showed better classification accuracy than the described methods.

5 Discussion

This paper focuses on channel selection for efficient classification of MI task in the BCI applications. In this work, we used ICA for special filtering, wavelet energy function for feature extraction and finally the extracted features are evaluated by three classifiers, LDA, SVM and KNN. This study investigates which electrode channels provide better performance with less computation cost. To build up an effective BCI system, it is important that we only use the electrodes that give the best accuracy. The finding of this study demonstrate that three channels named C3, C4 and Czare suitable channels for providing better motor imagery information from EEG data.

Acknowledgment. The authors thank Fraunhofer FIRST, Intelligent Data Analysis Group (Klaus-Robert Müller, Benjamin Blankertz), and Campus Benjamin Franklin of the Charité - University Medicine Berlin, Department of Neurology, Neurophysics Group (Gabriel Curio) for providing the data set.

References

1. Kamousi, B., Liu, Z., He, B.: Classification of motor imagery tasks for brain-computer interface applications by means of two equivalent dipoles analysis. IEEE Trans. Neural Syst. Rehabil. Eng. **13**(2), 166–171 (2005)
2. Wolpaw, J.R., et al.: Brain–computer interfaces for communication and control. Clin. Neurophysiol. **113**(6), 767–791 (2002)
3. Blankertz, B., et al.: The Berlin brain–computer interface: accurate performance from first-session in BCI-naive subjects. IEEE Trans. Biomed. Eng. **55**(10), 2452–2462 (2008)
4. Pfurtscheller, G., et al.: EEG-based discrimination between imagination of right and left hand movement. Electroencephalogr. Clin. Neurophysiol. **103**(6), 642–651 (1997)
5. Popescu, F., et al.: Single trial classification of motor imagination using 6 dry EEG electrodes. PLoS ONE **2**(7), e637 (2007)
6. Lim, C.-K.A., Chia, W.C.: Analysis of single-electrode EEG rhythms using MATLAB to elicit correlation with cognitive stress. Int. J. Comput. Theory Eng. **7**(2), 149 (2015)
7. Phinyomark, A., Chusak, L., Pornchai, P.: Optimal wavelet functions in wavelet denoising for multifunction myoelectric control. ECTI Trans. Electr. Eng. Electron. Commun. **8**(1), 43–52 (2010)
8. Oh, S.-H., Lee, Y.-R., Kim, H.-N.: A novel EEG feature extraction method using Hjorth parameter. Int. J. Electron. Electr. Eng. **2**(2), 106–110 (2014)
9. Resalat, S.N., Saba, V.: A study of various feature extraction methods on a motor imagery based brain computer interface system. Basic Clin. Neurosci. **7**(1), 13–20 (2016)
10. Yang, B.-H., et al.: Feature extraction for EEG-based brain–computer interfaces by wavelet packet best basis decomposition. J. Neural Eng. **3**(4), 251 (2006)
11. Shan, H., et al.: EEG-based motor imagery classification accuracy improves with gradually increased channel number. In: 2012 Annual International Conference of the IEEE Engineering in Medicine and Biology Society. IEEE (2012)
12. Blankertz, B., et al.: The BCI competition 2003: progress and perspectives in detection and discrimination of EEG single trials. IEEE Trans. Biomed. Eng. **51**(6), 1044–1051 (2004)
13. Siuly, S., Li, Y., Wen, P.: Modified CC-LR algorithm with three diverse feature sets for motor imagery tasks classification in EEG based brain computer interface. Comput. Methods Programs Biomed. **113**(3), 767–780 (2014)
14. Siuly, S., Li, Y., Wen, P.: Comparisons between motor area EEG and all-channels EEG for two algorithms in motor imagery task classification. Biomed. Eng. Appl. Basis Commun. (BME) **26**(3), 1450040 (2014). 10 pages
15. Siuly, Y.L., Wen, P.: Identification of motor imagery tasks through CC-LR algorithm in brain computer interface. Int. J. Bioinform. Res. Appl. **9**(2), 156–172 (2013)
16. Pfurtscheller, G., et al.: Mu rhythm (de) synchronization and EEG single-trial classification of different motor imagery tasks. Neuroimage **31**(1), 153–159 (2006)

17. Hyvärinen, A., Oja, E.: Independent component analysis: algorithms and applications. Neural Netw. **13**(4), 411–430 (2000)
18. Erfani, A., Abbas, E.: The effects of mental practice and concentration skills on EEG brain dynamics during motor imagery using independent component analysis. In: 26th Annual International Conference of the IEEE Engineering in Medicine and Biology Society (IEMBS 2004), vol. 1. IEEE (2004)
19. Wang, S., James, C.J.: Extracting rhythmic brain activity for brain-computer interfacing through constrained independent component analysis. Comput. Intell. Neurosci. **2007**, 9 (2007). Article ID 41468
20. Ting, W., et al.: EEG feature extraction based on wavelet packet decomposition for brain computer interface. Measurement **41**(6), 618–625 (2008)
21. Lotte, F., Guan, C.: Regularizing common spatial patterns to improve BCI designs: unified theory and new algorithms. IEEE Trans. Biomed. Eng. **58**(2), 355–362 (2011)
22. Baziyad, A.G., Ridha, D.: A study and performance analysis of three paradigms of wavelet coefficients combinations in three-class motor imagery based BCI. In: 2014 5th International Conference on Intelligent Systems, Modelling and Simulation. IEEE (2014)
23. Siuly, S., Li, Y., Zhang, Y.: EEG Signal Analysis and Classification: Techniques and Applications. Health Information Science. Springer, New York (2016). https://doi.org/10.1007/978-3-319-47653-7
24. Zarei, R., He, J., Siuly, S., Zhang, Y.: A PCA aided cross-covariance scheme for discriminative feature extraction from EEG signals. Comput. Methods Programs Biomed. **146**, 47–57 (2017)
25. Siuly, S., Li, Y.: Improving the separability of motor imagery EEG signals using a cross correlation-based least square support vector machine for brain computer interface. IEEE Trans. Neural Syst. Rehabil. Eng. **20**(4), 526–538 (2012)
26. Siuly, S., Li, Y.: Discriminating the brain activities for brain–computer interface applications through the optimal allocation-based approach. Neural Comput. Appl. **26**(4), 799–811 (2014)
27. Kabir, E., Siuly, S., Zhang, Y.: Epileptic seizure detection from EEG signals using logistic model trees. Brain Inform. **3**(2), 93–100 (2016)
28. Siuly, S., Kabir, E., Wang, H., Zhang, Y.: Exploring sampling in the detection of multicategory EEG signals. Comput. Math. Methods Med. **2015**, 1–12 (2015). Article ID 576437
29. Kabir, E., Siuly, S., Cao, J., Wang, H.: A computer aided analysis scheme for detecting epileptic seizure from EEG data. Int. J. Comput. Intell. Syst. **11**(1), 663–671 (2018)
30. Siuly, S., Li, Y.: Designing a robust feature extraction method based on optimum allocation and principal component analysis for epileptic EEG signal classification. Comput. Methods Programs Biomed. **119**(1), 29–42 (2015)
31. Siuly, S., Yin, X., Hadjiloucas, S., Zhang, Y.: Classification of THz pulse signals using two-dimensional cross-correlation feature extraction and non-linear classifiers. Comput. Methods Programs Biomed. **127**, 64–82 (2016)
32. Supriya, S., Siuly, S., Zhang, Y.: Automatic epilepsy detection from EEG introducing a new edge weight method in the complex network. Electron. Lett. **52**(17), 1430–1432 (2016)
33. Siuly, S., Wang, H., Zhuo, G., Zhang, Y.: Analyzing EEG signal data for detection of epileptic seizure: introducing weight on visibility graph with complex network feature. In: ADC 2016: Databases Theory and Applications, pp. 56–66

Data Management, Data Mining, and Knowledge Discovery Mining

Mining Medical Periodic Patterns
from Spatio-Temporal Trajectories

Dongzhi Zhang, Kyungmi Lee(ID), and Ickjai Lee(✉)(ID)

Discipline of Computer Science and Information Technology, College of Science
and Engineering, James Cook University, PO Box 6811, Cairns, QLD 4870, Australia
dongzhi.zhang@my.jcu.edu.au, {joanne.lee,ickjai.lee}@jcu.edu.au

Abstract. A spatio-temporal trajectory captures the movement behaviors of an object, and reveals various periodic patterns for the object such as where and when the object regularly visits. Due to the recent advances in GPS-enabled data collection devices such as mobile phones, a large set of spatio-temporal trajectories has been collected and available for analysis. These spatio-temporal trajectories could be used to identify those people who periodically visit medical centres for treatments (patients), working (health professionals) or other purposes. Spatio-temporal periodic pattern mining is to find periodic patterns for a certain place at regular intervals from spatio-temporal trajectories. Past studies attempt to find periodic patterns in medical contexts through time-series datasets, but not from spatio-temporal trajectories. In this study, we introduce a medical periodic pattern mining framework that utilises spatio-temporal periodic pattern mining approaches to find medical periodic patterns. We test the feasibility and applicability of our framework through a real-world publicly available dataset. Experimental results reveal that our framework is able to identify those people who regularly visit medical centres from those not, and also find medical periodic patterns revealing interesting medical behaviors.

1 Introduction

A trajectory represents a trail of movements. A spatio-temporal trajectory means the trajectory is spatially located and temporally recorded, and it exhibits a series of movements of an object (or a user). With rapid developments in GPS-enabled data collection devices such as mobile phones, a large number of GPS-collected spatio-temporal trajectories has been available, and mining spatio-temporal trajectories has become an important area of research [12]. It provides a new opportunity to analyse the behavior of moving object, and it is a solid candidate to identify those people who regularly visit medical centres for treatments (patients) and for working (health professionals). For instance, if a person who periodically visits a medical centre at 11am every Tuesday for a month could be seen as a patient whilst if a person who regularly comes to the medical centre at 9am everyday could be a health professional working in the place.

© Springer Nature Switzerland AG 2018
S. Siuly et al. (Eds.): HIS 2018, LNCS 11148, pp. 123–133, 2018.
https://doi.org/10.1007/978-3-030-01078-2_11

Spatio-temporal periodic pattern mining [12,14,16] is to find periodic patterns from spatio-temporal trajectories. These trajectories are typically noisy and irregularly sampled, and spatio-temporal periodic pattern mining must implement an effective preprocessing stage to make them suitable for data mining. Spatio-temporal periodic pattern mining could identify who are health and medical centre related personnel such as patients or health professionals using their corresponding trajectories, and to find medical periodic patterns that reveal valuable medical behaviours. Existing studies in periodic pattern mining can be classified into two categories. One is general periodic pattern mining and the other is spatio-temporal periodic pattern mining. The former includes periodic pattern mining in event/sequence [4,10], time series [2,7,9,11,21,24,27,28] and social networks data [8,19] whilst the latter involves spatio-temporal trajectories [3,12,14–16,25]. Past studies in periodic pattern mining in medical contexts fall in the first category. They mine periodic patterns from health time series datasets [2,7,11], and fail to mine medical patterns from spatio-temporal trajectories. Recent advances in spatio-temporal periodic pattern mining [25,26] enable us to handle irregularly sampled and noisy GPS-collected trajectories. In this paper, we propose a medical periodic pattern mining framework that utilises cutting-edge spatio-temporal periodic pattern mining approaches to identify a set of trajectories that exhibits periodic visits to medical centres, and also find medical periodic patterns.

Main contributions of this paper are:

- to propose a medical periodic pattern mining framework from spatio-temporal trajectories;
- to utilise cutting-edge spatio-temporal periodic pattern mining to identify a set of trajectories (possibly patients and health professionals) exhibiting periodic visits to medical centres;
- to find medical periodic patterns from spatio-temporal trajectories;
- to provide experimental results with a real world dataset, Geolife[1].

The rest of paper is organised as follows. Section 2 briefly reviews periodic pattern mining in medical contexts, and cutting-edge spatio-temporal periodic pattern mining. Section 3 introduces a medical periodic pattern mining framework and Sect. 4 displays comparative experimental results. Section 5 concludes and presents directions for future work.

2   Literature Review

In this study, we use the term a spatio-temporal trajectory to describe a set of recorded GPS positions and time stamps for an object or user. It is in a form of triplet (lon, lat, t) where (lon, lat) presents a 2D spatial location, lon is longitude and lat is latitude, whilst t represents a corresponding time stamp. A spatio-temporal trajectory is a set $T = \{(x_1, y_1, t_1), (x_2, y_2, t_2), ..., (x_n, y_n, t_n)\}$,

---

[1] https://privamov.github.io/accio/reference/datasets/.

such that $t_i < t_{i+1}$ for all $i \in \{1,...,n\}$, each (x_i, y_i, t_i) is a trajectory node (a GPS sample point) at time t_i, and $|t_{j+1} - t_j| \neq |t_{k+1} - t_k|$ for $\exists\, j, k$ where $1 \leq j \neq k \leq n$. Note that, T is irregularly sampled due to bad weather conditions, device malfunctions, GPS errors or unforeseen reasons.

Existing studies for periodic pattern mining can be divided into two groups: general periodic pattern mining and spatio-temporal periodic pattern mining. In the former, [4,10] mine periodic patterns in event/sequence data, and [2,7,9,11,27] focus on periodic patterns from time series data. Past studies in periodic pattern mining in medical contexts are based on time series datasets [2,7,11]. [11] proposes a method to find frequent occurring diseases in specific geographical area at a given time period using Apriori-based technique. [2] applies time annotated sequences to discover associative frequent patterns for describing trends of different biochemical variables along the time dimension. [7] applies fuzzy cognitive maps (FCMs) to extract medical concepts from temporal diabetes data for mining periodic frequent patterns. One common drawback with these approaches is that they deal with time series data considering the temporal dimension, but fail to consider the spatial dimension that indicates 'where' periodic patterns occur. In data-rich medical settings, it is important to effectively find which trajectory (user movement) is stopping at and visiting to medical centres, and what are their medical periodic patterns. For instance, a user 'A' is visiting to a clinic at 10am for an hour every morning for a period of one month could indicate the user 'A' has a regular medical treatment everyday for a month to cure a certain disease. Past studies with time series data cannot find this kind of spatiality associated periodic pattern.

The latter spatio-temporal periodic pattern mining is a solid candidate to detect these spatial and temporal associated periodic patterns. Several studies have been proposed in the field [3,12,14–16,25,26]. These studies can be classified into three sub-categories: (1) the fixed period approach; (2) the reference spot approach; and (3) the semantics-based approach. The fixed period approach [3,5] mixes bottom-up and top-down mining techniques to mine periodic patterns based on a user-provided fixed period. This approach first divides a long trajectory into sub trajectories by a user-specified period, and then applies a traditional density-based clustering DBSCAN [6] to cluster trajectory nodes to find dense regions, and allocates class labels to these generated dense regions. This approach is not fully exploratory and fails to detect periodic patterns with various periods. One additional limitation is that it is not straightforward to apply this approach to irregularly sampled trajectories. The reference spot approach [14,16] consists of three phases: (1) reference spots detection; (2) corresponding period detection for each reference spot; and (3) mining periodic patterns for each reference spot. This approach uses the Kernel-based method [23] to find reference spots that are frequently visited by moving objects, and use a combination of Fourier transform and autocorrelation [1,22] to detect a period for each reference spot. Finally, periodic behaviors are calculated by retrieving all the reference spots which are associated with corresponding period based on Kullback-Leibler Divergence [13]. The authors extended this work to handle trajectories with missing data using linear interpolation and movement prediction [17]. One major issue with this approach is that it handles spatiality and temporality separately, that is it fails to treat both spatiality and temporality simultaneously and equally. Another drawback is that this approach assumes regularly sampled trajectories, thus it is not suitable for irregularly sampled GPS-collected spatio-temporal trajectories. To overcome these drawbacks, [25] proposes an algorithm, Traclus (spatio-temporal) based on a spatio-temporal trajectory clustering to mine periodic patterns. Traclus (spatio-temporal) considers both spatiality and temporality at the same time in order not to miss any spatio-temporal aggregations, and their associated periodic patterns. The semantics-based approach [26] attempts to overcome these drawbacks from traditional spatio-temporal periodic pattern mining. This approach utilises semantic information extracted from background maps, identifies spatially and temporally aggregated dense regions from irregularly sampled trajectories, applies Hidden Markov Model (HMM) to identify semantically meaningful stops (places where an object or a user stays more than a user-specified threshold indicating the object or user is doing a meaningful behaviour such as medical treatment, surgery and consultation), apply Lomb-Scargle periodogram [18,20] to find periods for each semantically meaningful stop, and finally mine periodic patterns for each stopping place. The semantics-based approach is able to handle irregularly sampled trajectories and thus a solid candidate for this study.

3   Medical Periodic Pattern Mining Framework

Figure 1 depicts an overall framework of our medical periodic pattern mining from spatio-temporal trajectories. The framework first takes a set of GPS-collected spatio-temporal trajectories, and utilises two spatio-temporal periodic pattern mining approaches [25,26] to identify a subset of trajectories that periodically visit medical centres, and their corresponding medical periodic patterns. In this study, a modified version of [25] for medical periodic pattern mining is referred to as a spatio-temporal dominant approach whilst that of [26] is referred to as a semantics-dominant approach in this paper. Please refer to [25,26] for detailed processes.

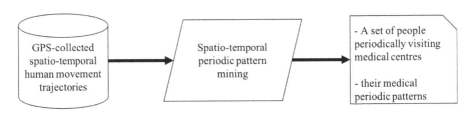

Fig. 1. Overall framework of medical periodic pattern mining from spatio-temporal trajectories.

Algorithm 1 shows a modified spatio-temporal dominant approach for medical periodic pattern mining whilst Algorithm 2 displays a modified semantics-dominant approach. Lines 8–11 in Algorithms 1 and 2 extract reference spots that contain medical centres for our study.

Algorithm 1. Spatio-temporal Dominant Approach

INPUT: A spatio-temporal trajectory $Traj$, $(\langle x_1, y_1, t_1 \rangle, \langle x_2, y_2, t_2 \rangle, \ldots, \langle x_m, y_m, t_m \rangle, \ldots, \langle x_n, y_n, t_n \rangle$, and a set $M = \{m_1, \ldots, m_k\}$ of medical centres;

OUTPUT: A set of medical periodic patterns;

1: /* make spatio-temporal trajectory with regular time interval */
2: Employ Linear interpolation to get the trajectory with a regular time interval, $t_i - t_{i-1} = t_j - t_{j-1}$ for $i \neq j \in \{1, \ldots, n\}$;
3: /* Find reference spots */
4: Extend Traclus to additional three implicit trajectory properties $\langle$Direction, Speed, Time$\rangle$ to find reference spots $R = \{r_1, r_2, \ldots, r_j\}$;
5: /* Extract medical centres from background maps */
6: Build M from background semantic maps;
7: /* Detect periods */
8: **for** each reference spot $r_i \in R$ **do**
9:     **if** r_i contains any $m_j \in M$ **then**
10:         Detect periods for each reference spot r_i, and store the periods in T_i;
11:     **end if**
12: **end for**
13: /* Find periodic patterns */
14: **for** each $t \in T_i$ **do**
15:     $p_t = \{p_i \mid t \in T_i\}$;
16:     Construct a symbolised sequence Q using p_t;
17:     Mining periodic patterns from Q;
18: **end for**

---

4 Experimental Results

4.1 Dataset

We use a real GPS dataset from Geolife that was collected from (Microsoft Research Asia) Geolife project by 182 users in a period of over five years (from 4/2007 to 8/2012) in Beijing, China. The dataset shows users' outdoor movements, including regular entertainment behaviours, shopping activities, and also visits to medical centres. Figure 2(a) displays two representative datasets: one in red recorded from 26/9/2008 to 10/10/2008 has periodic visits to medical centres (referred to as positive trajectory in this paper) whilst the other in black recorded from 25/10/2008 to 10/11/2008 does not have periodic visits to medical centres (referred to as negative trajectory). A set of medical centres in the study region is shown in Fig. 2(b).

Algorithm 2. Semantics Dominant Approach

INPUT: A spatio-temporal trajectory $Traj$, and a set M of medical centres;
OUTPUT: A set of periodic patterns with associated places;
    /* Find stopping places using HMM */
2: Find stop episodes $S = \{s_1, s_2, ..., s_n\}$;
    /* Map matching those stopping episodes to real places */
4: **for** each $s_i \in S$ **do**
      Match each stop episode in S to places $P = \{p_1, p_2, ..., p_n\}$;
6: **end for**
    /* Detect periods for each stopping place */
8: **for** each place $s_i \in P$ **do**
      if s_i contains any $m_j \in M$ **then**
10:      Detect periods for p_i that matches with s_i, and store the periods in T_i;
      end if
12: **end for**
    /* Mine periodic patterns */
14: **for** each $t \in T_i$ **do**
      $p_t = \{p_i \mid t \in T_i\}$;
16:      Construct a symbolised sequence Q using p_t;
      Mining periodic patterns from Q;
18: **end for**

4.2 Reference Spots for Positive and Negative Trajectories

Positive trajectories having periodic visits to medical centres are of interest in this paper. Thus, only reference spots for the red positive trajectory shown in Fig. 2(a) is analysed here as an example. In this paper, we use a time interval of 10 seconds to interpolate irregularly sampled raw trajectories for the

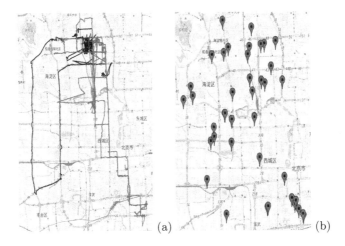

Fig. 2. Visualisations of two user trajectories and medical centres: (a) two spatio-temporal trajectories; (b) locations of medical centres.

spatio-temporal dominant approach. Table 1 shows that the semantic dominant approach can obtain more reference spots than the spatio-temporal dominant approach for the positive trajectory in study.

Table 1. Number of reference spots for the positive trajectory in red shown in Fig. 2(a).

Approach	Number of reference spots
Spatio-temporal dominant approach	9
Semantic dominant approach	16

4.3 Medical Periodic Patterns for Positive Trajectories

In this section, we present medical periodic patterns using both algorithms, and attempt to infer movement behaviors. Although the spatio-temporal dominant approach does not take background semantic information into account in the process of reference spot detection, we can post-match detected reference spots to nearest medical centres. Figure 3(a) displays 9 reference spots for the positive trajectory shown in Fig. 2(a) whilst Fig. 3(b) displays 10 reference spots for the negative trajectory using the spatio-temporal dominant approach. The 9 reference spots for the positive trajectory contain medical centres exhibiting frequent visits to medical centres whilst the 10 reference spots for the negative trajectory do not intersect with medical centres.

Figure 4 shows obtained reference spots for the positive trajectory in Fig. 2(a) using the semantic dominant approach. The arrows and numbers indicate i-th reference spots. Figure 4(b) and (c) show zoomed areas for the blue circle and red circle in Fig. 4(a), respectively.

Table 2 shows identified periodic patterns for the positive trajectory shown in Fig. 2(a) using the spatio-temporal dominant approach. As mentioned earlier,

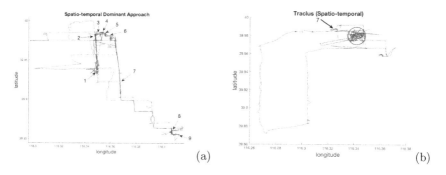

Fig. 3. Obtained reference spots for the positive trajectory and negative trajectory shown in Fig. 2(a) using the spatio-temporal dominant approach: (a) the positive trajectory; (b) the negative trajectory.

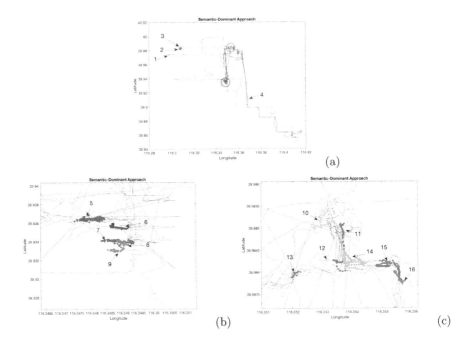

Fig. 4. Obtained reference spots for the positive trajectory shown in Fig. 2(a): (a) using the semantic dominant approach; (b) zoomed areas for the blue circle; (c) zoomed areas for the red circle. (Color figure online)

Table 2. Periodic patterns for the positive trajectory using the spatio-temporal dominant approach.

Reference spot	Period (Hours)	Periodic patterns
8	2	$9 \rightarrow 0 \rightarrow 8$
7	9	$6 \rightarrow 0 \rightarrow 7$

this method fails to take background semantic information into account, thus detected reference spots are not necessarily matched with medical centres. In this case, two periodic patterns detected are shown in Table 2. Since the spatio-temporal dominant approach focuses on finding periodic paths, reference spots 6–9 do not necessarily match with the medical centres shown in Fig. 2(b). For the periodic pattern $9 \rightarrow 0 \rightarrow 8$ and $6 \rightarrow 0 \rightarrow 7$, reference spots 6–9 are parts of roads as shown in Fig. 3. Thus, the spatio-temporal approach is not well suited for medical periodic pattern mining for our study.

Table 3 shows that obtained periodic patterns using the semantic dominant approach. In Table 3, a medical pattern, Peking University People's Hospital $6 \rightarrow 0 \rightarrow$ Building 5, shows a periodic pattern from reference spot 6 (Peking University People's Hospital) to reference spot 5 (Building 5). Reference spot 5 (a building) has a period of 8 h, which means the user goes to reference spot 5

Table 3. Periodic patterns for the positive trajectory using the semantic dominant approach.

Reference spot	Period (Hours)	Periodic patterns
Building 5	8	Peking University Hospital 6→ 0 → Building 5
Building 15	3	0 → Building 15
Medical centre 14	23	Student dormitory → 0 → Medical centre 14

(Building 5) every 8 h. 0 means the moving object is not in any reference spot. Another periodic pattern is reference spot 13 → 0 → reference spot 14, where reference spot 14 is matched to a medical centre whilst reference spot 13 is a student dormitory. This medical periodic pattern shows the user goes to the medical centre from the student dormitory periodically with a period of 23 h. In addition, 0 → reference spot 15 presents a periodic pattern for reference spot 15 (a building) with a period of 3 h.

Based on these periodic patterns, we can infer this user's health-related movement behaviors. There are two possible inferences: (Peking University People's Hospital 6→ 0 → Building 5) this user needs a periodic medical treatment at Peking University People's Hospital and goes to Building 5 at a period of 8 h. The user might have a treatment for few hours at hospital and comes back to Building 5 for resting; (Student dormitory → 0 → Medical centre 14) this person could be a student living in a student's dormitory, he/she needs to go to a medical centre regularly at a period of 23 h. The student might need to have a light treatment everyday at the medical centre.

To sum up, the semantic dominant approach is able to classify a user's movement (trajectory) into a positive trajectory or a negative trajectory, and also it finds medical periodic patterns for the positive trajectory. These medical periodic patterns could be used for hypothesis generation or further inference analysis.

5 Conclusion

A spatio-temporal trajectory captures a user's movements and is a solid candidate for mining medical periodic patterns. In this paper, we introduce a periodic pattern mining based framework for medical pattern detection. We utilise two recent spatio-temporal periodic pattern mining approaches to find medical periodic patterns, and demonstrate the feasibility and applicability of the proposed framework in medical settings using a real-world spatio-temporal movement trajectory dataset. Experimental results reveal that the proposed method is able to classify a user's trajectory into a positive trajectory (frequently visiting medical centres) or a negative trajectory (not frequently visiting medical centres), and also able to detect medical periodic patterns for the positive trajectory. These detected medical periodic patterns can be used for hypothesis generation, cause-effect analysis, and other data mining processes. More experimental results with diverse datasets would further validate the robustness of our approach. The semantic dominant approach is a solid approach for our purpose, but this cold be further optimised by tightly incorporating semantic medical information into the algorithm.

References

1. Bar-David, S., Bar-David, I., Cross, P., Ryan, S.J., Knechtel, C.U., Getz, W.M.: Methods for assessing movement path recursion with application to African Buffalo in South Africa. Ecology **90**(9), 2467–2479 (2009)
2. Berlingerio, M., Bonchi, F., Giannotti, F., Turini, F.: Mining clinical data with a temporal dimension: a case study. In: IEEE 2007 IEEE International Conference on Bioinformatics and Biomedicine, pp. 429–436 (2007)
3. Cao, H., Mamoulis, N., Cheung, D.W.: Discovery of periodic patterns in spatiotemporal sequences. IEEE Trans. Knowl. Data Eng. **19**(4), 453–467 (2007)
4. Cao, H., Cheung, D.W., Mamoulis, N.: Discovering partial periodic patterns in discrete data sequences. In: Dai, H., Srikant, R., Zhang, C. (eds.) PAKDD 2004. LNCS (LNAI), vol. 3056, pp. 653–658. Springer, Heidelberg (2004). https://doi.org/10.1007/978-3-540-24775-3_77
5. Cao, H., Mamoulis, N., Cheung, D.W.: Discovery of periodic patterns in spatiotemporal sequences. IEEE Trans. Knowl. Data Eng. **19**(4), 453–467 (2007)
6. Ester, M., Kriegel, H.P., Sander, J., Xu, X.: A density-based algorithm for discovering clusters in large spatial databases with noise. In: Proceedings of the 2nd International Conference on Knowledge Discovery and Data Mining, pp. 226–231. AAAI Press (1996)
7. Froelich, W., Wakulicz-Deja, A.: Mining temporal medical data using adaptive fuzzy cognitive maps. In: IEEE 2009 2nd Conference on Human System Interactions, pp. 16–23 (2009)
8. Halder, S., Samiullah, M., Lee, Y.K.: Supergraph based periodic pattern mining in dynamic social networks. Expert Syst. Appl. **72**, 430–442 (2017)
9. Han, J., Dong, G., Yin, Y.: Efficient mining of partial periodic patterns in time series database. In: Proceedings of the 15th International Conference on Data Engineering, pp. 106–115. IEEE Computer Society (1999)
10. Huang, K.-Y., Chang, C.-H.: Mining periodic patterns in sequence data. In: Kambayashi, Y., Mohania, M., Wöß, W. (eds.) DaWaK 2004. LNCS, vol. 3181, pp. 401–410. Springer, Heidelberg (2004). https://doi.org/10.1007/978-3-540-30076-2_40
11. Ilayaraja, M., Meyyappan, T.: Mining medical data to identify frequent diseases using Apriori Algorithm. In: IEEE 2013 International Conference on Pattern Recognition, Informatics and Mobile Engineering, pp. 194–199 (2013)
12. Jindal, T., Giridhar, P., Tang, L.A., Li, J., Han, J.: Spatiotemporal periodical pattern mining in traffic data. In: Proceedings of the 2nd ACM SIGKDD International Workshop on Urban Computing, UrbComp 2013, pp. 11:1–11:8. ACM, New York (2013)
13. Kullback, S., Leibler, R.A.: On information and sufficiency. Ann. Math. Statist. **22**(1), 79–86 (1951)

14. Li, Z., Ding, B., Han, J., Kays, R., Nye, P.: Mining periodic behaviors for moving objects. In: Proceedings of the 16th ACM SIGKDD International Conference on Knowledge Discovery and Data Mining, KDD 2010, pp. 1099–1108. ACM, New York (2010)
15. Li, Z., Han, J.: Mining periodicity from dynamic and incomplete spatiotemporal data. In: Chu, W.W. (ed.) Data Mining and Knowledge Discovery for Big Data. SBD, vol. 1, pp. 41–81. Springer, Heidelberg (2014). https://doi.org/10.1007/978-3-642-40837-3_2
16. Li, Z., Han, J., Ding, B., Kays, R.: Mining periodic behaviors of object movements for animal and biological sustainability studies. Data Min. Knowl. Discov. **24**(2), 355–386 (2011)
17. Li, Z., et al.: Movemine: Mining moving object data for discovery of animal movement patterns. ACM Transactions on Intelligent Systems and Technology **2**(4), 37 (2011)
18. Lomb, N.R.: Least-squares frequency analysis of unequally spaced data. Astrophys. Space Sci. **39**, 447–462 (1976)
19. Parthasarathy, S., Mehta, S., Srinivasan, S.: Robust periodicity detection algorithms. In: Proceedings of the 15th ACM International Conference on Information and Knowledge Management, CIKM 2006, pp. 874–875. ACM, New York (2006)
20. Scargle, J.D.: Studies in astronomical time series analysis. II - statistical aspects of spectral analysis of unevenly spaced data. Astrophys. J. **263**, 835–853 (12 1982)
21. Sheng, C., Hsu, W., Lee, M.L.: Mining dense periodic patterns in time series data. In: Proceedings of the 22nd International Conference on Data Engineering., p. 115. IEEE Computer Society (2006)
22. Vlachos, M., Yu, P., Castelli, V.: On periodicity detection and structural periodic similarity. In: Proceedings of the 5th SIAM International Conference on Data Mining, pp. 449–460 (2005)
23. Worton, B.J.: Kernel methods for estimating the utilization distribution in home-range studies. Ecology **70**(1), 164–168 (1989)
24. Yang, J., Wang, W., Yu, P.S.: Mining asynchronous periodic patterns in time series data. IEEE Trans. Knowl. Data Eng. **15**(3), 613–628 (2003)
25. Zhang, D., Lee, K., Lee, I.: Hierarchical trajectory clustering for spatio-temporal periodic pattern mining. Expert Syst. Appl. **92**, 1–11 (2018)
26. Zhang, D., Lee, K., Lee, I.: Semantic periodic pattern mining from spatio-temporal trajectories. Knowledge-Based Systems (2018, submitted)
27. Zhang, M., Kao, B., Cheung, D.W., Yip, K.Y.: Mining periodic patterns with gap requirement from sequences. ACM Transaction on Knowledge Discovery from Data **1**(2), 7 (2007)
28. Zhu, Y.L., Li, S.J., Bao, N.N., Wan, D.S.: Mining approximate periodic pattern in hydrological time series. In: Abbasi, A., Giesen, N. (eds.) EGU General Assembly Conference Abstracts. EGU General Assembly Conference Abstracts, vol. 14, p. 515, April 2012

Text Mining and Real-Time Analytics of Twitter Data: A Case Study of Australian Hay Fever Prediction

Sudha Subramani[1(✉)], Sandra Michalska[1], Hua Wang[1], Frank Whittaker[1], and Benjamin Heyward[2]

[1] Institute for Sustainable Industries and Liveable Cities,
Victoria University, Melbourne, Australia
{sudha.subramani1,sandra.michalska}@live.vu.edu.au
[2] Nexus Online Pty Ltd., Greenock, Australia

Abstract. Social media platforms such as Twitter contain wealth of user-generated data and over time has become a virtual treasure trove of information for knowledge discovery with applications in healthcare, politics, social initiatives, to name a few. Despite the evident benefits of tweets exploration, there are numerous challenges associated with processing such data, given tweets specific characteristics. The study provides a brief of steps involved in manipulation Twitter data as well as offers the examples of the machine learning algorithms most commonly used in text analysis. It concludes with the case study on the Australian hay fever prediction with the application of the selected techniques described in the brief. It demonstrates an example of Twitter real-time analytics for heath condition surveillance with the use of interactive visualisations to assist knowledge discovery and findings dissemination. The results prove the potential of social media to play an important role in meaningful results extraction and guidance for decision makers.

Keywords: Twitter · Machine learning · Text mining
Information retrieval · Knowledge discovery

1 Introduction

Twitter is one of the most popular social media websites, where users can post and interact via posts called 'tweets' and it has been growing hastily since its creation in 2006 [1]. The platform's enormous benefit is the short time span that the messages can reach wide network of users, playing major role in real-time analytics [2]. Due to its ease of use, speed and reach, Twitter became a platform to set trends and agendas in topics that range from healthcare, through politics, technology, stock market analysis and entertainment industry. As Twitter has become a source for collective wisdom, many research studies used this power to predicting real-world outcomes. Twitter is also a cost effective and less time-consuming than other information extracting techniques such as surveys and opinion polls.

© Springer Nature Switzerland AG 2018
S. Siuly et al. (Eds.): HIS 2018, LNCS 11148, pp. 134–145, 2018.
https://doi.org/10.1007/978-3-030-01078-2_12

The enormous and high volume of information that disseminates through millions of Twitter users accounts presents an interesting opportunity to obtain a meaningful insight into population behavioural patterns along with the prediction of future trends. Moreover, gathering information on how people converse regarding topic can assist many sectors in the real-world applications.

In terms of case study selected, nearly 1 in 5 Australians suffered from allergic rhinitis in 2014 to 2015 [3]. The forecasts do not look promising due to climate changes as well as new allergens, worsening air quality etc. As the meteorological data on an array of hay fever triggers is becoming more and more available, there is currently no equivalent for the estimates of its prevalence and severity at the fine-grained spatial and temporal level. Thus, the study was inspired to fill this gap by utilising the real-time, low-cost and freely available social media to develop a proxy for pollen allergy prevalence and explore potential associations with the environmental factors.

The remainder of the paper is organised as follows. Section 2 presents the brief overview of text mining for Twitter application. Section 3 discusses various preprocessing techniques while dealing with noisy and unstructured data. Section 4 presents different classification based algorithms used in text mining. Section 5 introduces the real-time analytics of Twitter data and its applications in various domains are discussed. Section 6 ends with conclusions.

2   Text Mining for Twitter Application

The unstructured or semi-structured language is commonly used on Twitter or any other social media platform. Hence, the various types of ambiguities occur, such as morphological, syntactic or semantic. People tend to ignore grammatical rules and spelling mistakes in their posts [4]. In recent years, social media has become an active research area that has drawn huge attention among the research community for information retrieval and abstract topics discovery. Nonetheless, the following characteristics of Twitter makes it challenging for that purpose:

1. Immense volume, fast arriving rate and short message restriction,
2. Large number of spelling and grammatical errors,
3. Use of informal and mixed language,
4. High content of irrelevant data.

Therefore, an extraction of meaningful information from such noisy data became complex problem to solve. Text mining intends to address the above-mentioned issues. Liu et al. [5] defined text mining as an extension of data mining to text data. Information retrieval, text analysis, clustering and natural language processing are the multidisciplinary fields in text mining techniques. They facilitate models based on interesting patterns development and assist predictability.

3   Pre-processing Steps in Text Analysis

During data collection, the unstructured text data contains a lot of challenges that make it particularly challenging to work with as described in previous section. At the same time, the pre-processing steps are essential in any subsequent analyses. Precisely, if the data is not cleaned properly, the text analysis techniques at the later stage simply leads to "garbage in garbage out" phenomena [6]. Even though the pre-processing consumes a great amount of time, it improves the final output accuracy [7]. Feature extraction and feature selection are two basic methods of text pre-processing.

The content of collected tweets varies from useful and meaningful information to incomprehensible text. The former contains people's opinion and relevant posts regarding the topic, whereas the latter may contain advertisements and it does not add value to the analysis. Hence, high quality information and features are extracted by incorporating some pre-processing techniques explained briefly in the following subsections.

3.1   Feature Extraction

The Feature Extraction can be further categorized as 3 methods such as Morphological analysis, Syntactical analysis and Semantic analysis. The 3 categories are briefly explained below. The feature extraction is used for many applications such as automatic tweets classification [8], opinion analyser [9] and sentiment classification [10].

Morphological Analysis. Morphological analysis deals mainly with tokenization, stop-words removal and stemming [7]. The tokenization is the process of breaking a stream of text into words or phrases called tokens. Stop word lists contain common English words like articles, prepositions, pronouns, etc. Examples are 'a', 'an', the', 'at' etc. Hasan saif et al. [11] investigated that removing stop words improves the classification accuracy in Twitter analysis by reducing data sparsity and shrinking the feature space. Stemming is used to identify the root of a word, to remove the suffixes related to a term and to save a memory space. For example, the terms 'relations', 'related', 'relates' can be stemmed to simply 'relate'. Different stemming algorithms are available in the literature, such as brute-force, suffix-stripping, affix-removal, successor variety, and n-grams [7]. Porter stemming [12] is applied to standardise terms appearance and to reduce data sparseness. In addition to the above 3 methods, non-textual symbols and punctuation marks are removed. Noisy tweets are filtered by eliminating links, non-ascii characters, user mentions, numbers and hashtags.

Syntactical Analysis. Syntactic analysis consists of Part-of-Speech tagging (POS-tagging) and parsing techniques [13]. It provides knowledge about grammatical formation of the sentence and it is used to interpret logical meaning from the sentence. The POS tagging defines contextually related grammatical sense in a sentence like noun, verb, adjective etc. Various approaches have been developed to implement POS tagging like Hidden Markov Model [13]. Parsing is another technique of syntactical analysis, where the sentence is represented in a tree-like structure and analysed for which group of words combine.

Semantic Analysis. Semantic analysis is the primary issue for relationship extraction form unstructured text [14]. This refers to wide range of processing techniques that identify and extract entities, facts, attributes, concepts and events to populate meta-data fields. This is usually based on two approaches like rule-based matching and machine learning approach. First approach is similar to entity extraction and requires the support of one or more vocabularies. Another one is machine learning approach and it deals with the statistical analysis of the content and derives relationship from the statistical co-occurrence of terms in the document corpus. WordNet-Affect [15] and SentiWordNet [16] are the popular approaches that are used to extract the useful contents from the textual message. Strapparava et al. [15] proposed the WordNet-Affect approach, a linguistic resource for a lexical representation of affective knowledge (affective computing is advancing as a field that allows a new form of human computer interaction in addition to the use of natural language). Another approach is SentiWordNet, which is proposed by Esuli et al. [16] and it is a publicly available lexical resource for opinion mining.

3.2 Feature Selection

Another essential step after feature extraction is feature selection that improves the scalability and accuracy of the classifier by constructing vector space. The main purpose of this approach is to select the most important subset of features from the original documents based on the highest score. The highest score is predetermined measure based on the importance of the word [17]. For the text mining, the high dimensionality of the feature space is the major hurdle, as it contains many irrelevant and noisy features. Hence Feature selection method is widely used to improve the accuracy and efficiency of the classifier. The selected features provide a good understanding of the data and retain original physical meaning.

A substantial amount of research has been applied to evaluate the predictability of features for the application in classification techniques. Among them, Peng et al. [18] studied how to select compact set of superior features at low cost according to a maximal statistical dependency criterion based on mutual information. Another approach is based on conditional mutual information and it is defined as a fast feature selection technique. This approach favours features that maximize their mutual information and ensures the selection of features that are both individually informative and 2-by-2 weakly dependent [19]. Mihalcea et al. [20] examined several measures to determine semantic similarity between short collections of text. It relies on simple lexical methods like pointwise mutual information and latent semantic analysis.

Another popular approach calculates feature vectors based on two basic methods, namely Term Frequency (TF) and Inverse Document Frequency (IDF). TF-IDF function is the combination of TF and IDF and is mainly used to estimate the frequency and relevancy of a given word in the document at the same time. Ramos et al. examined the results of applying TF-IDF to determine what terms in a corpus of documents might be more relevant to a query [21].

4   Literature Survey on Real-Time Analytics of Twitter Data

Twitter supports real time analytics in various aspects like spatial analytics, temporal analytics and text mining. Spatial analytics provides the visual representation of various trending topics across various geographical locations and temporal analysis presents an information about seasonal trends or outbreaks of various topics.

As for the examples, Kathy et al. [22] described a novel real-time flu and cancer surveillance system that uses spatial, temporal and text mining on Twitter data. The real-time analytics results are reported visually in terms of US disease surveillance maps, distribution and timelines of disease types, symptoms, and treatments. Several research studies focused on Twitter to analyse and predict sentiment analysis [23], opinion mining on political campaigns [24,25], natural disasters [26], epidemic surveillance [27], event detection [28], topic modeling [29–34], and so on. O'Connor et al. [25] and Tumasjan et al. [24] showed that sentiment analysis of tweets correlated with the voters' political preferences and closely aligned with the election results. Not only in the field of politics, but also in economics, have public tweets played a major role. Sentiment analysis has been previously studied on different aspects such as blogs and forums and has now been analysed in social media [35]. Bollen et al. [36,37] analysed that tweet sentiments can be used to predict trends of stock and it is directly correlated with them. Bruns et al. [38] and Gaffney et al. [39] observed that Twitter is a powerful tool to gather public opinion and create social change.

Sakaki et al. [26] investigated tweets during natural disasters and shown that it is able to detect earthquakes and send warning alerts to society. They considered each twitter user as a mobile sensor in Japan and the probability of an earthquake is computed using time and geolocation information of the user. Posting time and volume were modelled as exponential distribution to estimate locations of earthquake using kalman and particle filters. Their research further evidenced that earthquake can be sensed earlier than official broadcast.

Culotta et al. [40] analysed Twitter to detect influenza epidemic outbreaks that improves speed and cost reduction from traditional methods. Data of the user like gender, age and location can be used to provide more descriptive information about demographic insights compared to search queries. They detected influenza using multiple regression models and Quincey et al. [41] identified swine flu from Twitter using pre-defined keywords and terms co-occurrence method. These methods are analysed by searching the tweets with the keywords and detected anomalous change with the rapid flow in message traffic related to given keywords. The aids of such a method is to collect more focused information from the Twitter stream. Twitter proves to be an effective source to research in healthcare topics and analyse various diseases like cholera [27], cardiac arrest [42], alcohol use [43], tobacco [44], drug use [45], mood swings [46] and Ebola outbreak [47]. Michael et al. proposed a technique called Ailment Topic Aspect Model [48,49] to monitor the health care of public through the diseases, symptoms and treatments detection in tweets.

Hence, this section describes the real-time application of Twitter in various sectors like healthcare, politics, natural disasters, stock market analysis, sentiment analysis and so on.

5   Case Study of Australian Hay Fever Prediction from Twitter

5.1   Experiment

The case study aiming to utilise machine learning algorithms to estimate the prevalence of Hay Fever from Twitter data was conducted. The steps involved relevant tweets extraction, followed by the standard pre-processing tasks, manual annotation, automatic classification with logistic regression model, correlation with the external data sources and statistical validation.

The tweets were extracted during high pollen season (mid-August up till end-November 2017) in Australia (location bounding box in the extraction criteria) and included either the 'hay fever' or 'hayfever' related terms or one of the associated with this condition symptoms (according to Wikipedia [50]).

The dataset of 681 tweets was manually annotated by the author, producing 402 Hay Fever - HF (59% of dataset) and Non-Hay Fever tweets - N-HF (41% of dataset). The logistic regression classifier was selected to train and test the data with the 3-times repeated 5-fold cross-validation. The TF-IDF frequency function was applied and the feature selection using filter method was adopted. The uni-grams were used based on the Minimum term frequency threshold set heuristically to 10.

Next, the potential predictors such as the weather condition variables, common triggers of pollen allergies, were identified and daily observations were collected. These in turn were correlated with HF tweeting intensity in set of locations (8 major Australian cities) on each day covering the analysed period. The Pearson's correlation coefficients for each city and weather variable on a daily temporal level were produced. For spatial patterns discovery and real-time analytics the interactive maps were developed.

5.2   Results

The first step after tweets extraction and pre-processing was training the classifier to automatically identify HF tweets from the collected dataset. The accuracy obtained was 0.925 for 45 features based on the Minimum term frequency threshold of 10. Associated Kappa was 0.846.

Apart from high performance accuracy on a test dataset, the advantage of logistic regression classifier is an insight into the relevant terms used for prediction, thus allowing for any future selection criteria refinement. As the main goal is an overall system's sensitivity and precision maximisation, both extraction and classification form an integral part of a continuous improvement cycle.

The properly defined keywords allow to increase the ratio between the numbers of true positives to true negatives. Therefore, further investigation of terms identified as most predictive by the classifier and their corresponding coefficients enables better understanding of the classification criteria (Table 1). For instance, the word 'sneezing' was highly associated with HF related tweets, whereas 'allergy' occurred mostly in the false positives posts. Therefore, 'allergy' term is not recommended search query for future HF data extraction.

Table 1. Terms coefficients (shortlist).

Term	TF-IDF	Term	TF-IDF
Allergy	−2.47	Cat	−4.13
Reaction	0.82	Today	3.08
Sneezing	13.83	Itchy	0.74
Spring	2.74	Nose	1.83
Eye	0.23	Season	1.88

The words associations function further facilitated the knowledge discovery about the Hay Fever in Australia (Table 2). The combination 'watery eye' ($r = 0.46$) occurred with the correlation twice as high as either 'red eye' ($r = 0.23$) or 'swollen eye' ($r = 0.22$). The 'stuffy nose' ($r = 0.50$) was more common than 'itchy nose' ($r = 0.22$) and the 'sore throat' ($r = 0.46$) was the only meaningful and at the same time dominant association. The correlation score obtained is the degree of confidence in the word association. The values of the coefficients fall between 0.22 and 0.60 revealing moderate to strong correlation. The terms relevant to Hay Fever were underlined.

In terms of validation, the F test for the whole model proved statistically significant with $p < 0.001$. The highest adjusted r2 (adjusted for the number of predictors) was obtained for Melbourne (0.626). In other words, over 60% of the variance in the number of HF related tweets (as indicator of its prevalence) was able to be explained by the weather statistics and pollen data.

As pollen rates information for Melbourne covered only a proportion of the analysed period, the total number of observations included in the model was 67 (62.0% of the total). Regression constant was set to 0.

Finally, an interactive map to visually explore correlations of weather variables and HF tweeting intensity was developed. Strength and direction is

Table 2. Word associations and their corresponding correlation values for 'eye', 'nose' and 'throat' terms.

Eye		Nose		Throat	
Term	Correlation	Term	Correlation	Term	Correlation
watery	0.46	blow	0.6	sore	0.46
tired	0.31	bathroom	0.51	watery	0.32
itchy	0.3	stuffy	0.5	woke	0.3
red	0.23	hand	0.36	ear	0.26
drop	0.22	foundation	0.34	raw	0.26
barley	0.22	rub	0.34	thunderstorm	0.26
swollen	0.22	throat	0.25	heal	0.26
big	0.22	itchy	0.22	nose	0.25

Table 3. Multiple regression coefficients and p-values for Melbourne.

Statistic	Category	Unit	Completeness	Coef.	p-value
Min temperature	Temperature	Celsius	100.00%	−0.357**	0.045
Max temperature	Temperature	Celsius	100.00%	0.2	0.359
Ave temperature	Temperature	Celsius	100.00%	0.015	0.966
Rainfall	Precipitation	mm	100.00%	−0.156**	0.031
Evaporation	Precipitation	mm	100.00%	0.401***	0
Relative humidity	Precipitation	mm	100.00%	0.103***	0.007
Pressure	Pressure	hPa	100.00%	-0.007*	0.071
Max wind gust speed	Wind	km/h	100.00%	−0.037	0.334
Ave wind speed	Wind	km/h	100.00%	0.318***	0.001
Overcast	Overcast	oktas	100.00%	−0.296	0.162
Sunshine	Sunshine	hours	100.00%	−0.163	0.202
Pollen count	Pollen		62.00%	0.014	0.117

indicated by the size and colour gradient of the circle (orange indicates negative, whereas blue positive association) (Fig. 1).

5.3   Discussion

In terms of the analysis for Melbourne area, the moderately strong correlations were observed (Table 3). In particular, the positive correlation between the Average Wind Speed and HF tweeting pattern is worth noting as wind plays a major role in pollen grains spread, triggering the allergic symptoms. Another positive and significant correlation occurred for Evaporation and Relative Humidity. Usually, the plants are more likely to release their pollen into the air more on a sunny rather than rainy day. However, if the rain is occurring around a thunderstorm,

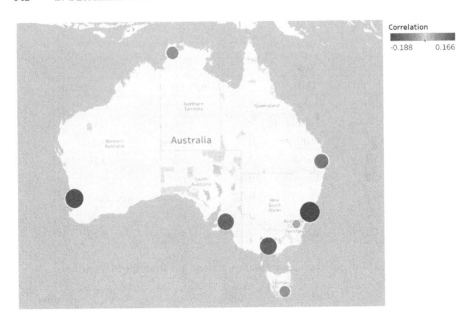

Fig. 1. Relative Humidity correlation map. (Color figure online)

then the humidity can make pollen grains burst open, releasing a high density of pollen into the air [51]. That may explain the coefficients values obtained. Furthermore, the Victoria State is known for its high probability of another co-related respiratory condition occurrence called thunderstorm asthma. As a matter of fact, the positive correlation for Relative Humidity variable paralleled the findings from the study on thunderstorm asthma predictability conducted in Melbourne reporting higher humidity with higher asthma admissions [52].

The correlation between pollen grains count and hay fever tweeting intensity was found insignificant (p = 0.117), although the value obtained was weakly positive (0.014). The pollen data for Melbourne was collected from 6 different pollen stations. In the analysis, the average was taken into account what might have affected the final output accuracy due to variations across the locations.

6   Conclusion

This survey provides the high-level overview of the specifics of Twitter data analysis, the challenges present as well as the current approaches to address them. The numerous applications utilising the real-time analytics potential from previous studies that transform unstructured tweets into valuable knowledge are given along with the case study on the Australian hay fever prediction. The experiment combined multiple heterogeneous data sources (numerical - structured vs text - unstructured) in order to obtain an instant insight into potential triggering factors of pollen allergy with the use of machine learning algorithms as well as interactive maps. The correlation values obtained allowed to measure the impact of specific variables in order to assist future forecasting ability. Finally, an analysis of logistic regression outputs (terms coefficients magnitudes and directions) enabled further extraction and classification criteria refinement for an on-going real-time analysis in a continuous improvement cycle.

References

1. Twitter. https://about.twitter.com/company
2. Bruns, A., Stieglitz, S.: Towards more systematic twitter analysis: metrics for tweeting activities. Int. J. Soc. Res. Methodol. **16**(2), 91–108 (2013)
3. Australian Institute of Health and Welfare. Allergic Rhinitis ('Hay Fever') in Australia (2016)
4. Sorensen, L.: User managed trust in social networking-comparing Facebook, Myspace and Linkedin. In: 1st International Conference on Wireless Communication, Vehicular Technology, Information Theory and Aerospace & Electronic Systems Technology, Wireless VITAE 2009, pp. 427–431. IEEE (2009)
5. Liu, F., Xiong, L.: Survey on text clustering algorithm-research present situation of text clustering algorithm. In: 2011 IEEE 2nd International Conference on Software Engineering and Service Science (ICSESS), pp. 196–199. IEEE (2011)
6. Dai, Y., Kakkonen, T., Sutinen, E.: MinEDec: a decision-support model that combines text-mining technologies with two competitive intelligence analysis methods. Int. J. Comput. Inf. Syst. Ind. Manag. Appl. **3**, 165–173 (2011)
7. Forman, G., Kirshenbaum, E.: Extremely fast text feature extraction for classification and indexing. In: Proceedings of the 17th ACM Conference on Information and Knowledge Management, pp. 1221–1230. ACM (2008)
8. Stavrianou, A., Brun, C., Silander, T., Roux, C.: NLP-based feature extraction for automated tweet classification. Interact. Data Min. Nat. Lang. Process. **145** (2014)
9. Zhao, P., Li, X., Wang, K.: Feature extraction from micro-blogs for comparison of products and services. In: Lin, X., Manolopoulos, Y., Srivastava, D., Huang, G. (eds.) WISE 2013. LNCS, vol. 8180, pp. 82–91. Springer, Heidelberg (2013). https://doi.org/10.1007/978-3-642-41230-1_7
10. Shirbhate, A.G., Deshmukh, S.N.: Feature extraction for sentiment classification on twitter data. Int. J. Sci. Res. (IJSR), 2319–7064 (2016). ISSN (Online)
11. Saif, H., Fernández, M., He, Y., Alani, H.: On stopwords, filtering and data sparsity for sentiment analysis of twitter (2014)
12. Porter, M.F.: Snowball: a language for stemming algorithms (2001)
13. Yuan, L.: Improvement for the automatic part-of-speech tagging based on Hidden Markov Model. In: 2010 2nd International Conference on Signal Processing Systems (ICSPS), vol. 1, pp. V1–744. IEEE (2010)
14. Jadhao, H., Aghav, D.J., Vegiraju, A.: Semantic tool for analysing unstructured data. Int. J. Sci. Eng. Res. **3**(8) (2012)
15. Strapparava, C., Valitutti, A., et al.: WordNet affect: an affective extension of WordNet. In: LREC, vol. 4, pp. 1083–1086. Citeseer (2004)
16. Esuli, A., Sebastiani, F.: SentiWordNet: a high-coverage lexical resource for opinion mining. Evaluation **17**, 1–26 (2007)

17. Montañés, E., Fernández, J., Díaz, I., Combarro, E.F., Ranilla, J.: Measures of rule quality for feature selection in text categorization. In: R. Berthold, M., Lenz, H.-J., Bradley, E., Kruse, R., Borgelt, C. (eds.) IDA 2003. LNCS, vol. 2810, pp. 589–598. Springer, Heidelberg (2003). https://doi.org/10.1007/978-3-540-45231-7_54

18. Peng, H., Long, F., Ding, C.: Feature selection based on mutual information criteria of max-dependency, max-relevance, and min-redundancy. IEEE Trans. Pattern Anal. Mach. Intell. **27**(8), 1226–1238 (2005)

19. Fleuret, F.: Fast binary feature selection with conditional mutual information. J. Mach. Learn. Res. **5**(Nov), 1531–1555 (2004)

20. Mihalcea, R., Corley, C., Strapparava, C.: Corpus-based and knowledge-based measures of text semantic similarity. In: AAAI, vol. 6, pp. 775–780 (2006)

21. Ramos, J., et al.: Using TF-IDF to determine word relevance in document queries. In: Proceedings of the First Instructional Conference on Machine Learning, vol. 242, pp. 133–142 (2003)

22. Lee, K., Agrawal, A., Choudhary, A.: Real-time disease surveillance using twitter data: demonstration on flu and cancer. In: Proceedings of the 19th ACM SIGKDD International Conference on Knowledge Discovery and Data Mining, pp. 1474–1477. ACM (2013)

23. Barbosa, L., Feng, J.: Robust sentiment detection on twitter from biased and noisy data. In: Proceedings of the 23rd International Conference on Computational Linguistics: Posters, Association for Computational Linguistics, pp. 36–44 (2010)

24. Tumasjan, A., Sprenger, T.O., Sandner, P.G., Welpe, I.M.: Predicting elections with twitter: what 140 characters reveal about political sentiment. Icwsm **10**(1), 178–185 (2010)

25. O'Connor, B., Balasubramanyan, R., Routledge, B.R., Smith, N.A.: From tweets to polls: linking text sentiment to public opinion time series. Icwsm **11**(122–129), 1–2 (2010)

26. Sakaki, T., Okazaki, M., Matsuo, Y.: Earthquake shakes twitter users: real-time event detection by social sensors. In: Proceedings of the 19th International Conference on World Wide Web, pp. 851–860. ACM (2010)

27. Chunara, R., Andrews, J.R., Brownstein, J.S.: Social and news media enable estimation of epidemiological patterns early in the 2010 Haitian Cholera outbreak. Am. J. Trop. Med. Hyg. **86**(1), 39–45 (2012)

28. Petrović, S., Osborne, M., Lavrenko, V.: Streaming first story detection with application to twitter. In: Human Language Technologies: The 2010 Annual Conference of the North American Chapter of the Association for Computational Linguistics, Association for Computational Linguistics, pp. 181–189 (2010)

29. Jiang, H., Zhou, R., Zhang, L., Wang, H., Zhang, Y.: A topic model based on Poisson decomposition. In: Proceedings of the 2017 ACM on Conference on Information and Knowledge Management, pp. 1489–1498. ACM (2017)

30. Huang, J., Peng, M., Wang, H., Cao, J., Gao, W., Zhang, X.: A probabilistic method for emerging topic tracking in microblog stream. World Wide Web **20**(2), 325–350 (2017)

31. Peng, M., Xie, Q., Wang, H., Zhang, Y., Tian, G.: Bayesian sparse topical coding. IEEE Trans. Knowl. Data Eng. (2018)

32. Peng, M., et al.: Mining event-oriented topics in microblog stream with unsupervised multi-view hierarchical embedding. ACM Trans. Knowl. Discov. Data (TKDD) **12**(3), 38 (2018)

33. Peng, M., et al.: Neural sparse topical coding. In: Proceedings of the 56th Annual Meeting of the Association for Computational Linguistics (Volume 1: Long Papers), vol. 1, pp. 2332–2340 (2018)

34. Yao, W., He, J., Wang, H., Zhang, Y., Cao, J.: Collaborative topic ranking: Leveraging item meta-data for sparsity reduction. In: AAAI, pp. 374–380 (2015)
35. Pang, B., Lee, L.: Opinion mining and sentiment analysis. Found. Trends® Inf. Retr. **2**(1–2), 1–135 (2008)
36. Bollen, J., Mao, H., Zeng, X.: Twitter mood predicts the stock market. J. Comput. Sci. **2**(1), 1–8 (2011)
37. Bollen, J., Mao, H., Pepe, A.: Modeling public mood and emotion: Twitter sentiment and socio-economic phenomena. Icwsm **11**, 450–453 (2011)
38. Bruns, A., Burgess, J.E.: # Ausvotes: How twitter covered the 2010 Australian federal election. Commun. Polit. Cult. **44**(2), 37–56 (2011)
39. Gaffney, D.: iranElection: quantifying online activism. In: Proceedings of the Web Science Conference WebSci10. Citeseer (2010)
40. Culotta, A.: Towards detecting influenza epidemics by analyzing twitter messages. In: Proceedings of the First Workshop on Social Media Analytics, pp. 115–122. ACM (2010)
41. de Quincey, E., Kostkova, P.: Early warning and outbreak detection using social networking websites: the potential of twitter. In: Kostkova, P. (ed.) eHealth 2009. LNICST, vol. 27, pp. 21–24. Springer, Heidelberg (2010). https://doi.org/10.1007/978-3-642-11745-9_4
42. Bosley, J.C., et al.: Decoding twitter: Surveillance and trends for cardiac arrest and resuscitation communication. Resuscitation **84**(2), 206–212 (2013)
43. Culotta, A.: Lightweight methods to estimate influenza rates and alcohol sales volume from twitter messages. Lang. Resour. Eval. **47**(1), 217–238 (2013)
44. Cobb, N.K., Graham, A.L., Byron, M.J., Niaura, R.S., Abrams, D.B., Participants, W.: Online social networks and smoking cessation: a scientific research agenda. J. Med. Internet Res. **13**(4) (2011)
45. Paul, M.J., Dredze, M.: Drug extraction from the web: Summarizing drug experiences with multi-dimensional topic models. In: Proceedings of the 2013 Conference of the North American Chapter of the Association for Computational Linguistics: Human Language Technologies, pp. 168–178 (2013)
46. Golder, S.A., Macy, M.W.: Diurnal and seasonal mood vary with work, sleep, and daylength across diverse cultures. Science **333**(6051), 1878–1881 (2011)
47. Odlum, M., Yoon, S.: What can we learn about the ebola outbreak from tweets? Am. J. Infect. Control. **43**(6), 563–571 (2015)
48. Paul, M.J., Dredze, M.: Discovering health topics in social media using topic models. PloS one **9**(8), e103408 (2014)
49. Paul, M.J., Dredze, M.: You are what you tweet: analyzing twitter for public health. Icwsm **20**, 265–272 (2011)
50. Allergic_rhinitis. https://en.wikipedia.org/wiki/Allergic_rhinitis
51. Allergy_cosmos. https://www.allergycosmos.co.uk/blog/why-is-my-hay-fever-worse-when-it-rains/
52. Silver, J.D., et al.: Seasonal asthma in Melbourne, Australia, and some observations on the occurrence of thunderstorm asthma and its predictability. PloS one **13**(4), e0194929 (2018)

A Data-Intensive CDSS Platform Based on Knowledge Graph

Ming Sheng[1(✉)], Qingcheng Hu[1], Yong Zhang[1], Chunxiao Xing[1],
and Tingting Zhang[2]

[1] RIIT&BNRCIST&DCST, Tsinghua University, Beijing 100084, China
`msheng24@126.com`,
`{huqingcheng,zhangyong05,xingcx}@tsinghua.edu.cn`
[2] Yellow River Engineering Consulting Co., Ltd., Zhengzhou 450000, China
`zhangtt@yrec.cn`

Abstract. Clinical Decision Support Systems (CDSSs) are very important for doctors and hospitals to improve the medical service quality. There are two types of CDSSs – knowledge-based CDSSs and data-intensive CDSSs. This paper presents a framework based on knowledge graph to integrate the two methods and proposes a data-intensive clinical decision support platform. This platform provides a series of clinical decision support services, including inquiry, inspection, diagnosis, medication & treatment and prognosis. This platform has been used in a system for village doctors.

Keywords: CDSS · Knowledge graph · Medical knowledge base
Data-intensive · Smart health

1 Introduction

Clinical Decision Support Systems (CDSSs) in Health Care have a long history going back to the 1970s. A CDSS is the computer software designed to contribute to clinical treatments and diagnoses [1]. More precisely, Clinical Decision Support (CDS) can be defined as "a process for enhancing health-related decisions and actions with pertinent, organized clinical knowledge and patient information to improve health and healthcare delivery", and a CDSS is an implementation of one or more CDS interventions [2]. CDSSs can support many different activities such as diagnosis, therapy, monitoring, or prevention and are used in all kinds of medical domains such as chronic illness, acute care, primary care, and patient advice lines. CDSSs may provide many different services such as access to knowledge, statistical calculations and individual adaptations, recommendations, reminders or alerts to different user groups.

There are two ways to facilitate the CDSSs: the knowledge-based systems and the data-intensive systems. The medical knowledge based systems perform a variety of functions, including knowledge acquisition, knowledge translation, logical reasoning based on evidence-based medical literature and the approved clinical practice guidelines. While the data intensive systems utilize the data from patients' Electronic Medical Records (EMR). Compared to medical knowledge based way, data-intensive way yields a significant performance overhead.

© Springer Nature Switzerland AG 2018
S. Siuly et al. (Eds.): HIS 2018, LNCS 11148, pp. 146–155, 2018.
https://doi.org/10.1007/978-3-030-01078-2_13

Through collaborating with hospitals, we have already put many efforts to apply big data and machine learning technologies to deal with health-related data. In [3], a deep learning based information extraction framework is designed to extract medical entities and relations from Chinese EMR. In [4], for the problem of patient's cost profile estimation, a model based on a patient's historical visits in EMR is presented. In [5], several deep learning algorithms are proposed to classify the topics of documents in diabetics. In [6], we investigate the influences of different language models on the sentiment classifications for Chinese health forums. In [7], a QA prototype is developed to answer health related questions. Based on these efforts, we decided to implement a system to integrate them to help doctors and hospitals.

This paper provides a unified framework based on knowledge graph to integrate knowledge-based and data-intensive methods, and designs a data-intensive clinical decision support platform - IDS. It follows the process of a patient's visit. This platform provides a series of clinical decision support services including inquiry, inspection, diagnosis, medication & treatment and prognosis.

This paper is organized as follows. Section 2 introduces the related work. Section 3 provides the integration framework. Section 4 presents the architecture of IDS. Section 5 shows the process of a patient visit in IDS. Section 6 demonstrates the application of IDS. Finally we conclude the paper in Sect. 7.

2   Related Work

In this section, we will discuss the related work from three aspects: knowledge-based CDSSs, data-intensive CDSSs and the application of CDSSs.

Knowledge-Based CDSSs: Shen et al. [8] described the construction and optimization of the sensitivity and specificity of a decision support system named IDDAP, which is based on ontologies for infectious disease diagnosis and antibiotic therapy. Nazari et al. [9] utilized expert systems and fuzzy logic, and developed an intelligent system, which is capable of diagnosing occurrence of heart diseases. Ohno-Machado [10] considered the update of medical knowledge base and the contextual information.

Data-Intensive CDSSs: In [11], a Semantic Web-based, multi-strategy reasoning approach is presented and integrates deductive and plausible reasoning and exploits Semantic Web technology to solve complex clinical decision support queries. Beaudoin et al. [12] evaluated the machining learning for CDSS to enhance antimicrobial stewardship programs. Piri et al. [13] analyzed data from more than 1.4 million diabetics and developed a CDSS for predicting DR.

Application of CDSSs: Greenes et al. [14] discussed how to integrate workflow-oriented models with a user-interactive mode of CDSS. Huberts et al. [15] introduced an innovative structured modeling approach in which model personalization is guided by sensitivity analysis and in which the effect of input uncertainties and model assumptions are considered during model corroboration. Humm et al. [16] described a personalised CDSS for cancer care. Anya et al. [17] presented the design of an awareness environment for cross-boundary clinical decision support in e-health that takes account of the concept of work practice as a design requirement. Bennett et al. [18] provided a substantive review of international literature evaluating the impact of CDSSs on the care of emergency department (ED) patients. Wajid et al. [19] discussed some of the current challenges in designing an efficient CDSS as well as some of the latest techniques that have been proposed to meet these challenges.

Our method combines these two strategies - knowledge-based method and data-intensive method, and will be discussed detailly in the next section

3 Integration Framework

Current CDSSs use either the knowledge-based method or the data-intensive method. There are few works to consider them together. This paper designs a new integration framework which could combine these two methods together.

The simplest way is to use them separately in one system. For a decision problem, if there are enough features in the input data, the knowledge-based method will be used. Otherwise, the data-intensive method will be used. These two methods can also be used at the same time, thus the final output will be the weighted average of the outputs from them.

In the knowledge-based method, the foundation is the medical knowledge base. While in the data-intensive method, the foundation is the medical sample base. The key to combine these two methods is how to connect the medical knowledge base and the medical sample base.

We propose a unified framework to connect the medical knowledge base and the medical sample base. Base on this framework, the medical knowledge base can be expanded and the medical sample base can be improved as well. So that the decision support efficiency can be improved. Specifically, it includes two aspects:

- The medical sample base supports the medical knowledge base: Based on a large number of samples, the framework can discover new rules and even discover problems within the original rules, so that the medical knowledge base can be constantly expanded and verified.
- The medical knowledge base supports the medical sample base: The relationships between the features of one sample are very important, which can contribute to both the selection of learning models and the adjustment of their parameters. Those relationships between features may be revealed by the medical knowledge base.

In order to support the above two aspects, we use the knowledge graph as a link between the medical sample base and the medical knowledge base. Specifically, we extract the triples from the medical sample base to form a knowledge graph. We perform rule detection in the knowledge graph, abstract those rules into knowledge and add them to the medical knowledge base. Meanwhile, we could apply the medical knowledge base to the knowledge graph, i.e., we can give more semantics to the nodes and edges as well as create more connections between the nodes. Moreover, those semantics and connections can be mapped to the relationships among the features of the data from the medical sample base.

4 Platform Architecture

Guided by the integration framework, we developed IDS - a data-intensive clinical decision support platform, whose architecture is shown in Fig. 1. It has eight modules: data integration (①), knowledge fusion (②), medical sample base (③), medical knowledge graph (④), medical knowledge base (⑤), model integration (⑥), rule reasoning (⑦) and IDS services (⑧).

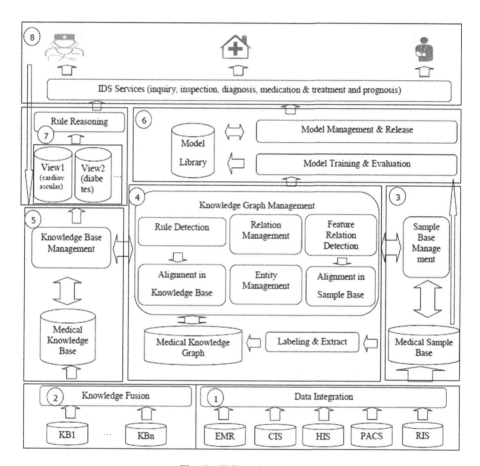

Fig. 1. IDS Architecture

The main functions of IDS are described below:

- Data integration: It includes four parts: the raw data storage, the data standard management, the data cleaning and the data management.
- Knowledge fusion: Based on the open knowledge bases in various fields and the international mainstream standards such as ICD10, this module performs knowledge fusion on various knowledge repositories.

- Medical sample base: It standardizes the records from the data integration and models those records based on the knowledge graph.
- Medical knowledge graph: It includes rule detection, relation management, feature relation detection, alignment in medical knowledge base, entity management, alignment in medical sample base and labeling & extract.
- Medical knowledge base: It includes code management, metathesaurus management, semantic network management, specialist lexicon management, and new concept/relation review.
- Model integration: It includes model training, model management and model release. The whole process includes model selection, model training, model evaluation, parameter tuning and model persistence. All of the models are stored in the model library.
- Rule reasoning: For certain specific area such as cardiovascular and diabetes, it performs a rule reasoning based on customized views from the medical knowledge base.
- IDS Services: It packs the selected models from model management & release module. With the packed models, the platform will provide web services that follow restful standards. It includes chief complaint input formalization, intelligent diagnosis, disease-based intelligent recommendation, similar case matching, rehospitalization risk prediction.

5   The Process of a Patient Visit in IDS

Around the process of a patient visit, this platform provides a series of clinical decision support services - inquiry, inspection, diagnosis, medication & treatment and prognosis. This process is based on the models which are trained by the data from the medical sample base, or the rules in the medical knowledge base (see Fig. 2). Due to page limit, here we only discuss the implementation based on model integration.

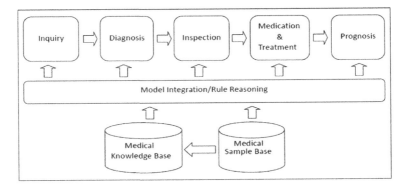

Fig. 2. The process of IDS

5.1 Inquiry

This step includes two functions. The first one is to help doctors regulate their chief complaints and remind doctors of key information that is easy to ignore (see Table 1). The second one is to match the most similar case according to the chief complaint.

Table 1. Chief complaint input formalization.

Input (Voice input) :
My name is Zhang San, male, 85 years old. Suffering from continuous chest tightness at about 9:00 pm three days ago and feeling dyspnea and arrhythmia. At the same time I also feel nauseous and sweating, vomiting, and numbness in the upper extremities. There has been no sign of remission.

Output:
[Sex]: (male)
[Age]: (85)
[Weight]: (unkown)
[First symptoms]: (persistent chest tightness) (stomach ache) (difficulty breathing)
[Concomitant symptoms]: (nausea) (vomiting) (upper limb numbness)
[Onset nature]: (persistent)
[Incentives]: (unkown)
[The longest duration of chest pain]: (unkown)
[Mitigation mode]: (can't ease)
[Past history]: (unkown)
The "unknown" part is a reminder to the doctor so that the doctor can further inquire.

5.2 Diagnosis

(1) Intelligent diagnosis. The input of this function is the structured chief complaint data, and the output is disease risk ranking, e.g.:

1. [ACS cardiogenic chest pain 80%]:
    1.1 (STEMI 60%)
    1.2 (Aortic dissection 20%)
2. [Non-ACS cardiogenic chest pain 15%]:
    2.1 (Arrhythmias 10%)
    2.2 (Ischemic cardiomyopathy 5%)
    2.3 (Coronary heart disease xx%)
3. [Non-cardiogenic diseases 5%]:
    3.1 (Respiratory diseases 3%)
    3.2 (Digestive system diseases 1%)
    3.3 (Nervous system disease 1%)

(2) Cardiovascular diseases risks ranking. The input of this function is the dynamic or static image files and the output is the disease risk ranking.
(3) Similar case matching. The input of this function is the structured chief complaint, inspection result and diagnosis. The output is based on the EMR from hospitals that is stored in the medical sample base, as described above.

5.3 Inspection

(1) Intelligent inspection items recommendation. The input of this function is the disease risk ranking and the output is the suggested inspection e.g.:

[Sign detection]:
(blood oxygen xx%) (blood pressure xxx/xxx mmHg) (ECG)
[Blood test]:
(creatinine xx umol/L) (BNP xx pg/ml) (PT-INR x) (creatinine protein xx ng/ml)

(2) Similar case matching. The input of this function includes the structured chief complaint and inspection result. The output is based on the EMR from hospitals that is stored in the medical sample base.

5.4 Medication and Treatment

(1) Intelligent medication & treatment recommendation. The input of this function is the structured chief complaint, diagnostic result and inspection result. The output is the medication and medical treatment advice, e.g.:

Medication advice:
[Ant platelet]: (Aspirin)
[Anti-angina]: (Nitroglycerin)
[Sedative]: (Morphine)
[Heart rate, blood pressure]: (Atropine) (Dopamine)
[Surgical treatment]: (Interventional surgery)
Medical treatment advice:
[Conventional disposal]: (CPR) (Oxygen absorption) (Defibrillation)
[Surgical treatment]: (Interventional surgery)
[Unable to dispose of]: (Enter a high level of specialist treatment)

(2) Similar case matching. The input of this function contains the structured chief complaint, diagnostic result and inspection result. The output is based on the EMR from hospitals that is stored in the medical sample base, as described above.

5.5 Prognosis

After going through the whole process of a patient visit (inquiry, inspection, diagnosis, medication & treatment), this platform provides the prognosis prediction services. The purpose is to assess the effectiveness of treatment from the perspective of health economics. Specifically this platform uses re-hospitalization risk prediction model to achieve the above purpose. Meanwhile the input of the service is just like the EMR from hospitals which is stored in the medical sample base. The output of the service is the days of re-hospitalization.

6   Application of IDS

6.1   Motivation

At present, the quality of primary health care in China is at a relatively low level. Many village doctors need professional guidance from experienced doctors who are very busy themselves. CDSS could help village doctors to reduce their misdiagnosis rate. We applied IDS to support the village doctors.

6.2   Implementation

The application was developed using Hadoop, Spark, Scale and Java. Figure 3 shows an example of decision support for diagnosis. The input of this interface contains three parts:

1. The upper left part of the figure is the chief complaint input area, such as sex, age and weight.
2. The lower left part of the figure is the current medical history input area which is text input.

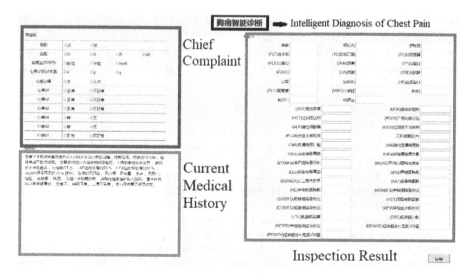

Fig. 3.   Example of User Input Interface

3. The right part of the figure is the inspection result input area, such as blood oxygen, blood pressure, creatinine, BNP, PT-INR and creatinine protein.

The output is disease risk ranking (see Fig. 4).

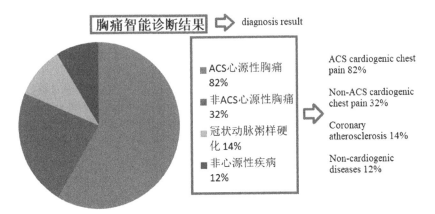

Fig. 4. Example of Result Interface

7   Conclusion

This paper proposes IDS, a data-intensive clinical decision support platform based on knowledge graph. This paper designs a new integration framework which connects the medical knowledge base and the medical sample base. Under this framework, the medical knowledge base can be expanded and the medical sample base can be improved as well. Therefore, the decision support efficiency can be improved. Following the process of a patient visit, this platform provides a series of clinical decision support services. The platform has been integrated in an application for village doctors.

References

1. Berner, E.S.: Clinical Decision Support Systems: Theory and Practice, vol. 233. Springer, New York (2007). https://doi.org/10.1007/978-0-387-38319-4
2. Osheroff, A., Teich, J.M., Levick, D.: Improving Outcomes with Clinical Decision Support: An Implementer's Guide, 2nd edn. Healthcare Information and Management Systems Society (HIMSS), Chicago (2012)
3. Tian, B., Zhang, Y., Liu, K.X., Xing, C.X.: Deep learning based information extraction framework on Chinese electronic health records. In: SEKE, pp. 86–91 (2018)
4. Zhao, K., et al.: Modeling patient visit using electronic medical records for cost profile estimation. In: Pei, J., Manolopoulos, Y., Sadiq, S., Li, J. (eds.) DASFAA 2018. LNCS, vol. 10828, pp. 20–36. Springer, Cham (2018). https://doi.org/10.1007/978-3-319-91458-9_2

5. Chen, X., Zhang, Y., Zhao, K., Hu, Q., Xing, C.: Domain supervised deep learning framework for detecting Chinese diabetes-related topics. In: Pei, J., Manolopoulos, Y., Sadiq, S., Li, J. (eds.) DASFAA 2018. LNCS, vol. 10828, pp. 53–71. Springer, Cham (2018). https://doi.org/10.1007/978-3-319-91458-9_4

6. Zhang, Y., Zhang, Y., Xu, J., Xing, C., Chen, H.: Sentiment analysis on Chinese health forums: a preliminary study of different language models. In: Zheng, X., Zeng, D.D., Chen, H., Leischow, Scott J. (eds.) ICSH 2015. LNCS, vol. 9545, pp. 68–81. Springer, Cham (2016). https://doi.org/10.1007/978-3-319-29175-8_7

7. Yin, Y., Zhang, Y., Liu, X., Zhang, Y., Xing, C., Chen, H.: HealthQA: a Chinese QA summary system for smart health. In: Zheng, X., Zeng, D., Chen, H., Zhang, Y., Xing, C., Neill, Daniel B. (eds.) ICSH 2014. LNCS, vol. 8549, pp. 51–62. Springer, Cham (2014). https://doi.org/10.1007/978-3-319-08416-9_6

8. Shen, Y., Yuan, K.: An ontology-driven clinical decision support system (IDDAP) for infectious disease diagnosis and antibiotic prescription. Artif. Intell. Med. **86**, 20–32 (2018)

9. Nazari, S., Fallah, M., Kazemipoor, H., Salehipour, A.: A fuzzy inference- fuzzy analytic hierarchy process-based clinical decision support system for diagnosis of heart diseases. Expert Syst. Appl. **95**, 261–271 (2018)

10. Ohno-Machado, L.: Clinical decision support: informatics interventions for better patient care. JAMIA **25**(5), 457 (2018)

11. Mohammadhassanzadeh, M., Woensel, W.V., Abidi, R.S.: Semantics-based plausible reasoning to extend the knowledge coverage of medical knowledge bases for improved clinical decision support. BioData Min. **10**(1), 7:1–7:31 (2017)

12. Beaudoin, M., Kabanza, F., Nault, V.: Evaluation of a machine learning capability for a clinical decision support system to enhance antimicrobial stewardship programs. Artif. Intell. Med. **68**, 29–36 (2016)

13. Piri, S., Delen, D., Liu, T.: A data analytics approach to building a clinical decision support system for diabetic retinopathy: Developing and deploying a model ensemble. Decis. Support Syst. **101**, 12–27 (2017)

14. Greenes, R.A., Bates, D.W., Kawamoto, K., Middleton, B.: Clinical decision support models and frameworks: seeking to address research issues underlying implementation successes and failures. J. Biomed. Inform. **78**, 134–143 (2018)

15. Huberts, W., Heinen, S.G.H., Zonnebeld, N.: What is needed to make cardiovascular models suitable for clinical decision support? A viewpoint paper. J. Comput. Sci. **24**, 68–84 (2018)

16. Humm, B.G., Walsh, P.: Personalised clinical decision support for cancer care. In: Hoppe, T., Humm, B., Reibold, A. (eds.) Semantic Applications, pp. 125–143. Springer, Heidelberg (2018). https://doi.org/10.1007/978-3-662-55433-3_10

17. Anya, O., Tawfik, H.: An "Awareness" environment for clinical decision support in e-health. In: Rojas, I., Ortuño, F. (eds.) IWBBIO 2018. LNCS, vol. 10814, pp. 456–467. Springer, Cham (2018). https://doi.org/10.1007/978-3-319-78759-6_41

18. Bennett, P., Hardiker, N.R.: The use of computerized clinical decision support systems in emergency care: a substantive review of the literature. JAMIA **24**(3), 655–668 (2017)

19. Wajid, S.K., Hussain, A., Luo, B., Huang, K.: An investigation of machine learning and neural computation paradigms in the design of clinical decision support systems (CDSSs). In: Liu, C.-L., Hussain, A., Luo, B., Tan, K.C., Zeng, Y., Zhang, Z. (eds.) BICS 2016. LNCS (LNAI), vol. 10023, pp. 58–67. Springer, Cham (2016). https://doi.org/10.1007/978-3-319-49685-6_6

Analysing the Impact of Electronic Health Records

Ziheng Wang[(⊠)]

Information System, School of Engineering, The University of Melbourne,
Melbourne, Australia
wzhwalter@gmail.com

Abstract. This paper aims to analyse the impact of the national electronic health records. It focuses on private health insurance market, business process re-engineering, and other considerations. It uses principles of microeconomic, business process, and dynamic management with examples to predict possible situations during system implementation.

Keywords: Electronic health records · Health insurance · Re-engineering

1 Introduction

According to the report, *Realizing the Full Potential of Health Information Technology to Improve Healthcare for Americans,* the information technology can improve the efficiency of the access to patient data, so the performance of medical work can and have benefit from information technology in health care environment [1]. A very typical implement is 'electronic health records', which aims to provide complete, valid, and real-time data of patients to clinicians, so that it improved the quality and reduce the time of diagnostic method and treatments. However, almost 80% of physicians lack even rudimentary digital records; and most of electronic health record is lack of the ability of interoperability [2].

Building an integrate electronic health record system is worth to consider because of considerable advantages. In this paper, it is going to analyse the macroscopical impact of the electronic health record system in the public rather than only focus on the how it influences hospital, clinic or patient [3].

2 Private Health Insurance Market

Except universe health insurance, some individuals are willing to purchase private health insurance from companies. The most common reason for having private insurance is security, protect and peace of mind (54.7%) in 2012 [4]. Health care costs can be unpredictable and very large [5]. In such a situation, people will want to purchase insurance. The insurance companies pool together individuals who are facing the similar risk of the health and aim to lower and eliminate the risk.

© Springer Nature Switzerland AG 2018
S. Siuly et al. (Eds.): HIS 2018, LNCS 11148, pp. 156–163, 2018.
https://doi.org/10.1007/978-3-030-01078-2_14

A very common issue in insurance market is asymmetric information. It exists when one party in a transaction has information that is not available to another party in the transaction [6]. If insurance companies cannot obtain the complete and valid information from the customer, they are difficult to identify and estimate the possibility of and economical loss of the 'getting sick'. In general, individuals with high health risk have incentive to hide part of their real health status to ask for a lower premium. Therefore, insurance company cannot charge the individual, who has a larger economical loss or high possibility of the getting sick, a higher premium. In this case, the individual has more information about their health, while insurance companies have less or invalid information. Therefore, the insurance companies have to charge an average premium which based on the population's health status to cover the unexpected payouts caused by the asymmetric information. In other word, because of the lack of information, insurances companies do not have ability to dividend different individual with different health level into to different categories. The population-based premium is expected to be higher for the individuals who has low risk and low expected loss; and be lower for the individuals who has high risk and expected loss.

Furthermore, the asymmetric information may cause further impacts. Some most common reason for individual not having private health insurance are 'can't afford it and too expensive'; 'lack of value for money/not worth it' [7]. The higher and expensive price of premium for some individuals can be partially explained by population-based estimation of risk that we discussed above. 'lack of value' means that individuals believe the utility gained by insurance in dollar is less than they paid for an insurance in dollar. Therefore, some individual, who have private insurance demand, have to exit the market, especially the individual group which have low possibility of risk, low economic loss of risk, and low level of risk aversion. Moreover, this phenomenon may cause the failure in insurance market. In the most extreme case, all individuals who have low risk exit the market, then the insurance collapses. The reason is that the insurance company cannot afford the expensive payout, because they charge an average population-based premium, but all remained individuals have expected high possibility of or high economic loss of the health risk. In general case, there will be still some individuals who has less health risk purchase the insurance, even the premium is not fair for them. The reason is that some individuals are high level of risk aversion. In other word, they are facing a greater loss of utility if they get sick, so they are willing to pay more money to release the loss caused by the risk. In this case, the market may not collapse, but this market is not efficiency.

These problems are examined by Cutler and Reber at Harvard University. Harvard employees could purchase a more general health insurance with a slightly higher price than if they purchase a less general health insurance [8]. The university changed the subsidy rule: university paid the same amount of subsidy to any of the insurance. Therefore, the price of the more general insurance is much more expensive than the price of the less general insurance at this time. Many employees decided to switch their insurance plan to less general one. These employees were relatively younger and were expected have a better health. The premium of the general insurance was doubled because the company had to cover the higher expected cost of the relatively older and less healthy population who remained in the general plan. The increased price led to more youngers leave the general insurance again. In the next year, the general insurance was dropped, so the market collapsed.

The problems we discussed above are caused by the root issue asymmetric information. These problems may be released by a national integrate electronical record system. The individual health information can exchange between government, hospital, and insurance company. The private company may not have authority to access the database of patient information or operate the system, but they can ask for a hard copy of the record from their customer who want to purchase the insurance. The authoritative record can provide a more complete, valid and reliable information of the individual; thus, insurance company will have a clear understanding of the individual's health status, and evaluate the risk properly based on this information. Risk evaluation may depend on variety variables, such as age, gender, job, medical history. Then, individuals can be divided into more proper category. Therefore, partial asymmetric information problems can be solved by the electronic record system. For example, individual is getting hard to hide their real health status to ask for a lower insurance premium. The overall market efficient will be improved.

However, the system enables the information accessible may cause problems. The premium of the high-level health risk is excepted too expensive for individual to afford it. Perhaps, it looks reasonable, but the there is a problem in how the risk is estimated. We do not have a perfect formula, or indicator to calculate the health risk [6]. For example, female group usually has a longer average life than male group, but it does not mean female A will have longer life than male B. However, in this situation, the insurance company may charge different premium to A and B. Some people will feel uncomfortable about the categories. Therefore, categories may raise some problems of price discrimination (Fig. 1).

	Hospital Type	Software Package	Result of the Implementation Process	People Interviewed
Case 1	Community hospital	Alpha	Failure	Physicians:7 Nurses:4 Mangers:5
Case 2	University hospital	Alpha	Success	Physicians:4 Nurses:4 Mangers:5

Fig. 1. Electronic Medical Records packages in two Canadian hospitals

3   Re-engineering of the Medical Process

The rapidly developed information technology paly an important role to increase the efficiency of the medical process. IT enables the original process executed in a totally different approach. It is not just seen IT as a tool to automate some tasks, we should use IT as an integral part of the overall business organization capital to redesign the aged process [7]. The business value of using IT is not from IT directly; it comes from the new efficient process. The process re-engineer is usually result in a large variation in scope and amount of the change in many projects, and it focuses on costing-cutting and downsizing [8].

Electronic health record system is not only automatically using IT to collect and save a bunch of digital patient health records [11–13]. It should be an integral part of the overall process because it may help the medical process executed in a totally different and efficient way. Consequently, it will bring a very large change of the medical process. The more efficient process is our aim, but only one in three large BPR projects was considered successful [14]. Even the same implement of IT in different places may bring different outcome. The management of the change is a key determination of the change process outcome: failure or success.

LaPointe and Rivard stated a very clear case of outcome influenced by resistance [15]. There are two same Electronic Medical Records packages were implemented in two Canadian hospitals, but brought two different outcomes. In both hospitals the goal was to computerize patient records, prescription systems. The diagrams show the situation of the hospitals and the resistance change in the project (Fig. 2).

In both cases, resistance initially exist. From doctor's aspect, the implement of the alpha package damages their utility: the system slowed them down because they have to enter information by themselves. Thus, doctors think they are ignored by the management, so the further resistance occurs. The different outcomes of two hospitals' result of different management's response. In case 1, the board believed the system is good, and the doctors are unnational, so the response lead to the further doctor's resistance. Eventually, the hospital might have to close because some doctors decided to resign, and resistance-level going up. Thus, the change project seems failure. In case 2, the management of the hospital considered carefully about the complaint letter send by the doctors, and finally they decided to relax the schedule of the project; also, they withdrew part of the package implement that cause the resistance of the doctor and developed the further improved system. After four years, the system was used by all hospital departments, so the project was success (Fig. 3).

A radical change of process usually accompanies with down-sizing, redundancy, creation of new roles or creation of new procedures. It is necessary to identify the impact of the change positively and negatively; who is stakeholders and why stakeholders are effect [16]. Success or otherwise will be reliant heavily on how well the stakeholders accept and use the new system as well as how much benefit the stakeholders sees in the outputs [16]. Moreover, the change can be emotionally draining; the Kubler-Ross model states the emotions in different stages. Therefore, for the electronic record system implement, not only the rational impact analysis should be considered

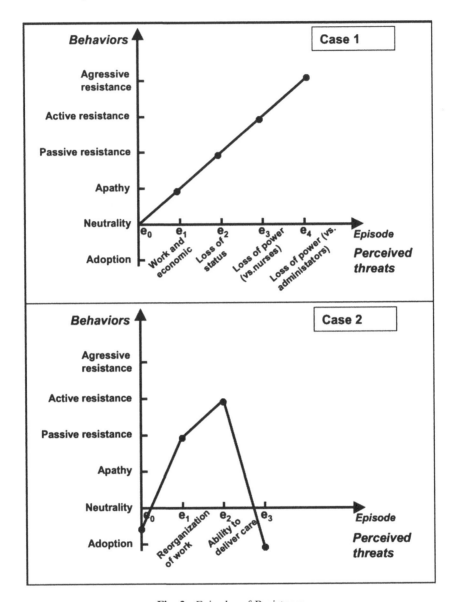

Fig. 2. Episodes of Resistance

carefully, but also the emotional problems of stakeholders should managed well to ensure the succeed of the project.

Change can be emotional

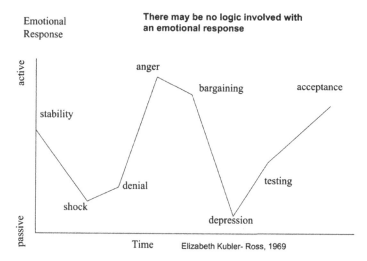

Fig. 3. Kubler-Ross model

4 Other Considerations

4.1 Government Health Expenditure

In 2013–14, governments were responsible for $105 billion, or nearly 68% of total health expenditure of $155 billion in Australia. The health expenditure occupied a large proportion of government expenditure around 16% in recent years [17]. The estimate health expenditure is important for government to control the budget not overrun. The integrate electronic record system can provide a complete and valid residents medical record to predict and estimate the cost of patient health care. Moreover, the large volume of data may help government understand the health level of the resident and evaluate the health demand of resident. Therefore, it may play an important role in the government health investment, such as hospital location choice, medical research project investment.

4.2 Database Administration Management

An integrate national electronic record system implies the large volume of data should be managed properly. It may be too difficult and costly to design a rational database for the big data, the records data should be exchanged between the different organizations and distributed in different regions. Thus, the initial cost is expected too expensive. Moreover, compare with financial data transaction, the consistency of the medical record is relatively not that important. Therefore, the expensive cost of a rational database may be not very suitable. However, rational database is very efficient to obtain and analyse the across subfields of aggregates. Thus, further research on health can benefit from this important attribute. Therefore, there is a trade between cost and efficiency at this point.

Security of the database is another issue accompanies with the global or national access of database [18–20]. Private information leaking is a serious social problem now, just like the Facebook event in this year. The public are more and more sensitive and nervous about their private information security [21, 22]. Some of them may reject to input their information into database [23]. Therefore, the security problem should be considered and released carefully to avoid further problems [24].

4.3 Other Externality

The electronic record aims to improve the efficiency and quality of the medical process [25, 26]. It may reduce the time-consuming of the health consulting, diagnose and surgery. So, it may contribute to reduce the patient's long waiting time. However, it brings a negative externality. A more efficient process really kind of affect medical staff's wellbeing. For example, a doctor meets 10 patients per day, but if the system faster the process, the doctor will meet 12 patients per day. Thus, the workload of the doctor increases, the doctor will feel uncomfortable about the system if there is no compensation (such as more salary) for the increased workload.

The increased quality of the medical process also brings positive externality. For example, if we can heal some patients with infectious diseases in short time, it reduces the possibility of other healthy people reflected by infectious diseases.

5 Conclusion

The paper illustrates some consideration and analysis of the possible impacts of an integrity electronical health record system implement in the society. There impacts can be negative either positive to the social welfare. Before the project eventually implement, the detailed evaluation of gain and loss based on the overall society should be analysed; and the benefit trade-off between different group should be judged carefully.

References

1. President's Council of Advisors on Science and Technology (PCAST): Executive Office of the President, Report to the President Realizing the Full Potential of the Health Information Technology to Improve Healthcare for Americans: The Path Forward (2010)
2. Kabir, E., et al.: A computer aided analysis scheme for detecting epileptic seizure from EEG data. Int. J. Comput. Intell. Syst. 11, 663–671 (2018)
3. Vimalachandran, P., et al.: The Australian PCEHR system: ensuring privacy and security through an improved access control mechanism. EAI Endorsed Trans. Scalable Inf. Syst. 3 (8), e4 (2016)
4. Australian Health Survey: Health service usage and health related actions, 2011–12. http://www.abs.gov.au/ausstats/abs@.nsf/lookup/E334D0A98272E4DCCA257B39000F2DCF?opendocument. Accessed 5 July 2018

5. Supriya, S., et al.: Weighted visibility graph with complex network features in the detection of epilepsy. IEEE Access **4**, 6554–6566 (2016)
6. Rosen, H., Wen, J., Snoddon, T.: Public finance in Canada, 4th edn, pp. 161–172. McGraw-Hill Ryerson Limited, USA (2012)
7. Harmon, P.: The scope and evolution of business process management. In: vom Brocke, J., Rosemann, M. (eds.) Handbook on Business Process Management 1, pp. 50–52. Springer, Berlin (2010). https://doi.org/10.1007/978-3-642-00416-2_3
8. Cutler, M., Sarah, R.: Paying for health insurance: the trade-off between competition and adverse selection. Q. J. Econ. **113**(2), 433–466 (1998)
9. Smith, W.: Why Processes Matter II: Efficiency (2018)
10. Siuly, S., et al.: Exploring sampling in the detection of multicategory EEG signals. Comput. Math. Methods Med. 10–22 (2015)
11. Li, M., et al.: Privacy-aware access control with trust management in web service. World Wide Web **14**(4), 407–430 (2011)
12. Thongkam, J., et al.: AdaBoost algorithm with random forests for predicting breast cancer survivability. In: IEEE International Joint Conference on Neural Networks (IEEE World Congress on Computational Intelligence), pp. 3062–3069 (2008)
13. Vimalachandran, P., et al.: Cryptographic access control in electronic health record systems: a security implication. In: Bouguettaya, A., et al. (eds.) WISE 2017. LNCS, vol. 10570, pp. 540–549. Springer, Cham (2017). https://doi.org/10.1007/978-3-319-68786-5_43
14. Nohria, N., Beer, M.: Cracking the Code of Change. Harvard Business Review (2000). https://hbr.org/2000/05/cracking-the-code-of-change. Accessed 5 July 2018
15. LaPointe, L., Rivard, S.: A multilevel model of resistance to information technology implementation. MIS Q. **29**(3), 461–491 (2005)
16. Mendoza, A: Change Management (2018)
17. Australian Institute of Health and Welfare: Australia's Health. Australia's health series no. 15. Cat. no. AUS 199. Australia Government, Canberra, p. 3 (2016)
18. Sun, L., et al.: Semantic access control for cloud computing based on e-Healthcare. In: 2012 IEEE 16th International Conference on Computer Supported Cooperative Work in Design (CSCWD) (2012)
19. Wang, H., et al.: A flexible payment scheme and its role-based access control. IEEE Trans. Knowl. Data Eng. **17**(3), 425–436 (2005)
20. Sun, X., et al.: Satisfying privacy requirements before data anonymization. Comput. J. **55**(4), 422–437 (2012)
21. Wang, H., et al.: Special issue on security and privacy of IoT. World Wide Web **21**(1), 1–6 (2018)
22. Sun, X., et al.: Publishing anonymous survey rating data. Data Min. Knowl. Discov. **23**(3), 379–406 (2011)
23. Zhang, J., et al.: Outlier detection from large distributed databases. World Wide Web **17**(4), 539–568 (2014)
24. Zhang, J., et al.: On efficient and robust anonymization for privacy protection on massive streaming categorical information. IEEE Trans. Dependable Secure Comput. **14**(5), 507–520 (2017)
25. Cohen, A., Siegelman, P.: Testing for adverse selection in insurance markets. J. Risk Insur. **77**(1), 39–84 (2010)
26. Sun, L., et al.: Purpose based access control for privacy protection in e-healthcare services. J. Softw. **7**(11), 2443–2449 (2012)

Development of New Architectures and Applications

Building Applications that Matter: Co-designing with Adolescents with Autism Spectrum Disorder

Randy Zhu$^{(\boxtimes)}$, Dianna Hardy , and Trina Myers

James Cook University, Queensland, Australia
{randy.zhu, dianna.hardy, trina.myers}@jcu.edu.au

Abstract. Technology-based applications for people with special needs are on the rise as mobile devices and wearable technology become more pervasive in society. However, the development of applications for special needs can be an intricate process due to the physical or mental challenges of the prospective users. Individuals with *Autism Spectrum Disorder* (ASD) process the world differently and often encounter poor *User Experience* (UX) with applications that are not designed with them in mind. Application design approaches should be inclusive and partner with users and communities to increase application acceptance, improve useable features and create enjoyable interfaces; yet this is not current software design practice. A pilot study was conducted to investigate how adolescents with ASD use technology and explore how they could participate as co-designers in the early phases of application development. Two co-design workshops were conducted with six adolescents with ASD over one month where they engaged in the application ideation and design phases of a software design process through the use of group discussion and drawings. This paper presents the results of the pilot study and discusses the role of ASD participants in co-designing software applications for wearable technology and how they felt about their involvement in the process. Key themes were identified by thematic analysis of the data collected. Preliminary data suggest that participants: (1) are technology savvy users; (2) experience poor UX due to their unique perceptive; and (3) expect to make design decisions for applications built for them.

Keywords: Co-design · Participatory design · Autism Spectrum Disorder
Human computer interaction · User experience

1 Introduction

Autism Spectrum Disorder (ASD) describes a range of neurodevelopmental disorders characterized by impaired social and communication development, repetitive behaviors and restricted interest [1, 2]. These challenges span the lifetime of those diagnosed, but early intervention for children diagnosed with ASD may result in an improvement in both their social and non-social challenges over time [3]. The current generation of adolescents are first class digital citizens, having had access to computers and technology as a part of their daily lives since early childhood. In addition, many adolescents

© Springer Nature Switzerland AG 2018
S. Siuly et al. (Eds.): HIS 2018, LNCS 11148, pp. 167–174, 2018.
https://doi.org/10.1007/978-3-030-01078-2_15

with ASD find technology to be engaging and prefer to access or use technology over other leisure and social activities. While the use of technology-based interventions or applications built for individuals with ASD is on the rise, not all applications are well received [4]. Failing to consider the unique perspectives of users with ASD can lead to a lack of uptake of technology.

Co-design is a methodological approach that includes all stakeholders who will be affected by the artifact, including both the users and their caregivers, in the design process. Co-design has been adopted in previous ASD research, specifically in developing software used for education or intervention. Due to co-design's emphasis on balancing power inequities, participants report feeling valued, safe and able to contribute meaningfully to the design process. This involvement can increase user "buy-in" and support the likelihood of an end product that is useful, usable and desirable [5].

A pilot study was conducted to investigate how adolescents with ASD use technology and to explore how these adolescents can participate as co-designers in the early phases of application development. This paper presents the results of the pilot study and discusses the role of ASD participants in the co-design process and how they felt about their involvement in co-designing software applications for wearable technology.

Two co-design workshops were conducted across a period of one month with six adolescents with ASD. Participants engaged three co-design roles (i.e., Learner, Mentee, and Partner) over the workshops to develop skills needed to contribute to the software design process. The research team (i.e. a combined group of both researcher and participants) completed the application ideation and design phases of a software design process through the use of group discussion and drawings. The researcher also acted as the software developer and developed the first prototype at the end of the second workshop. Finally, thematic analysis was applied to the data collected and three key themes were identified that included: (1) are technology savvy users, (2) experience poor *User Experience* (UX) due to their unique perceptive and (3) expect to make design decisions for applications built for them. Preliminary results from the pilot study serve as reference points for future workshops that will explore special needs software design and development.

2 Technology and Autism Spectrum Disorder

There were approximately 164,000 Australians (0.5%) with ASD in 2015, which shows a 42.1% increase from 2012 where 115,400 people were estimated to have the condition [6]. The number of individuals diagnosed with ASD in Australia is expected to continue to increase due to an elevated awareness of the condition, and improved diagnostic processes. Currently, there is no cure for ASD, however, customized interventions such as speech correction and cognitive, physical and motor skills therapies can lessen the deficits [3].

Symptoms of social skills challenges include: evasive eye contact, difficulty in interpreting verbal and nonverbal social cues, delayed or poor response towards social stimulus, inappropriate emotional response, and lack of empathy to others' distress [1, 2]. Despite these challenges, research has found that children diagnosed with ASD are able to better express themselves through the use of technology and have a higher tendency to interact with other ASD children when both are interested in the specific technology [7]. A study by Kuo et al. [8] focused predominantly on adolescents' media use and reported that 98% of the 92 participants with ASD used computers approximately five hours per day to watch cartoons and play games. In a similar study, Mazurek et al. [9] found that children (8–18) with ASD spent on average 4.5 h per day using screen-based media (i.e. video games and television) compared to 2.8 h per day in non-screen activities (playing with friends, engaging in sports and reading). These studies show that individuals with ASD have a strong interest in and preference for the use of technology in their day to day activities.

The ways we interact with computers has changed significantly with the introduction of smart devices. The wide proliferation of such devices has resulted in the reduction of barriers to entry such as affordable hardware and unified software development tool kits. These conditions propelled the creation of technology-based application development for individuals with disabilities. However, not all applications are well received by the intended users. The lack of understanding between users' needs and functionality, device availability, poor device performance, and change in user needs or priorities are significantly related to user frustration that can potentially lead to software abandonment [10].

An observational study on the use of iPad applications found that children and young adults with ASD were more productive in completing a desired task with the help of a professional guide [11]. In this comparative study, participants were observed in a classroom environment while using an iPad and data coding found that participants spent an average of 45% of the time "lost" in the application (difficulties in finding/following the steps to complete a task). In comparison, participants only spent an average of 16% of the time "lost" in the application when a guide is present [11]. A well-designed application should match the individual's specific needs, do the intended job for which it was designed and has an intuitive user interface [12]. Additionally, individuals need to view the device positively and be amenable to incorporate the use of the device into their activities. The use of co-design methods includes these considerations during all development phases in collaboration with the consumers and communities [13].

2.1 Co-design with Participants with Autism Spectrum Disorder

The use of co-design in software development can result in an improved UX, which relates to a person's overall attitudes and feelings about a product, system or service and how easy or pleasant that product is to use [10]. UX tests ensure that the user finds value in the use of a product [14]. In the co-design approach, the developer guides stakeholders through iterative phases of problem definition, solution ideation and prototype implementation via workshops with the aim to improve the UX [15].

Co-design workshops often use qualitative methods such as a design charrette (i.e. a design workshop) where users can discuss or communicate ideas through group discussion or drawings. The research teams use low-fidelity prototypes such as sketches and paper storyboards to frame requirements, generate ideas and test solutions in the workshops. This pragmatic approach allows the research team to learn and adjust the requirements of the end product through each cycle. The iterative workshops aim to incorporate human-centred design and activity-centred design, creating software that is applicable in their daily activities [16].

The co-design method has been adopted in previous ASD research, specifically in developing software used for education or intervention, due to its empathetic focus and collaborative nature. However, there have been differences in the level of participation from the stakeholders. Frauenberger et al. [17] suggest three categories of approach that included:

1. Non-participatory approaches: informed by theory, best practice or prior experience but having no direct involvement of, for example, children with autism.
2. Participation via proxy: those with intimate knowledge of the user population, such as parents and teachers, represent the needs of the children.
3. Full participation: defined as "any form of involvement that allows children with disabilities to have a direct impact on the outcome".

Most co-design based ASD research is conducted with participants in early childhood and adopts the participation via proxy approach where parents, carers or psychologists are involved in the design process instead of the children themselves. The participation via proxy approach is preferred when there are considerable challenges in communication, cognitive and behavioral difficulties [18]. However, the participation via proxy approach does not allow the individuals with ASD, who are the actual end-users of the software, to directly influence design decision. Studies show individuals with ASD expect to be included in design decisions that affects them and the risk of software abandonment can be reduced with user-involvement during the design and development [18]. A further study to develop a facial expression recognition software with adolescents with ASD found the use of co-design provides insights into the usability of a system and was critical to the development of a technology [19].

3   Observed Preliminary Results

Evidence from the literature suggests that adolescents with ASD may perceive application interfaces differently from others and their unique perception may influence the way they use technology. Francis et al. [18] found that individuals with ASD expect to be involved in design decisions and noted that more research needed to be conducted on appropriate methods.

This pilot study investigated how adolescents with ASD used technology and how they could contribute as co-designers in the early phases of application development. The research team consisted of the researcher/software developer and six adolescents with ASD recruited from the *North Queensland Autism Support Group* (NQASG). The pilot study included two workshops and was conducted across a period of one month. Participants are engaged in three co-design roles (1) Learner; (2) Mentee; and (3) Partner over the two workshops.

In the first workshop, the pilot study was introduced to the group by the researcher who led a group discussion through structured and unstructured questions related to their experience in using technological devices and software. Game design was chosen for the pilot study as participants are familiar with computer games and expressed interest in developing their own game. The first workshop engaged the participants as "Learner" and "Mentee" roles. The researcher trained the participants (Learner) in basic skills around game design (i.e. the use of drawings to illustrate ideas and levels) and encouraged the participants to design their own individual computer games. The researcher provided the participants (Mentee) one-to-one guidance on individual game design techniques in the final stage of this workshop.

The Partner role was the focus of the second workshop where the researcher formed a research team with the participants. The team were tasked to design a game of their interest and to produce a low-fidelity prototype (drawings) for the game. The research team expressed their ideas through group discussion and used drawings to illustrate ideas and game level design with one level for each section of the game. A low-fidelity paper prototype of the game was designed at the end of the session.

3.1   Findings

A thematic analysis identified three key themes and the results suggest that participants: (1) are technology savvy users, (2) experience poor UX due to their unique perceptive and (3) expect to make design decisions for applications built for them (Table 1). Participants are savvy technology users and are familiar with the latest gadgets and applications. Most of them use computers and mobile devices on a daily basis for education or leisure purposes. Participants also commented that they are familiar with navigating and downloading contents from Google Play Store and Apple App Store and use social media and YouTube to stay informed of the latest gadgets and games.

Table 1. Thematic analysis results.

Theme	Example participant quotes
Experience poor UX	*"I don't understand why some software took long to load up. I can't wait."* *"I like to upload my own YouTube videos but I just cannot remember the steps to do upload. Every time."*
Expect to make design decisions for applications built for them	*"I find it annoying to use an application with different fonts and colours."* *"I don't like to follow instructions on a computer, I just want it to show me what I like to do."* *"Now that I know how to design game, I want my game in my way."* *"My favourite colour is blue. I want the font colour to be this."* *"I only like to use the applications where I have interest in."* *"If I can change the layout, it will look very different and I think I will like it more."*

Participants highlighted frustrations with poor UX design. For example, the interface for applications such as YouTube (to upload videos) and educational software or games used at home or school seem difficult for them. The majority of the participants have very strong preferences in terms of user interface such as the font type, color and interface layout. One participant commented that he prefers text to be in blue even if the background is blue though having the same foreground and background colour tends to make text less readable and is generally avoided in user interface design.

Participants commented on the lack of input from people with ASD into applications that target them as users. They face difficulties using applications that are built specifically for them such as intervention or education applications. Participants found using applications to be difficult when the design does not consider their preferred interaction style and abilities. At the end of second workshop, participants commented that they feel more confident and comfortable in using an application where they can be involved in the design process.

Participants engaged in the discussion and were able to provide in-depth details of their preferences and experiences in terms of collaborating in a group. Despite their ASD challenges, participants were able to engage and communicate with peers and the researcher in regard to technology where they shared a common interest. Some participants initially did not actively engage in the group discussion and took a while to "warm up" to the environment. A number of participants preferred to use drawing to illustrate their ideas and message as compared to verbal communication.

4   Conclusions

Designing applications for people with special needs has always been a challenge in terms of application usability and usefulness [5]. This group of users are often locked out of the software design process by the lack of involvement in the design decisions and are often forced to accept applications that do not take their challenges in consideration [20]. An empathetic and inclusive design approach should be taken to ensure equal power relationships between designers and users for people with special needs [21].

The preliminary results of the pilot study presented in this paper show that adolescents with ASD are technology savvy users and in most cases, they prefer to use technology in their daily lives. Due to their ASD challenges, they may experience an application differently compared to their peers and in some cases, the inability to perform the task on an application could lead to user frustration. In addition, individuals with ASD may not have the means or ability to explicitly describe or feedback their user experience to the designers of applications, even when they are required to use them in everyday life. The preliminary results also show that participants with ASD when given the opportunity and equal balance of power, are able to engage actively in group discussion and contribute to the software design process.

Evidence from the pilot study suggests that the use of co-design in software design is an approach with great potential for people with ASD. However, an entire software design cycle needs to be completed to further investigate the effectiveness and inclusiveness of the co-design methods that involve individuals with ASD.

The results and outcomes from this pilot study will inform the second phase of this study that aims to co-design a smartwatch application with adolescents with ASD. The second phase will involve three rounds of an iterative software design process across seven workshops that include the research team (i.e. the researcher and participants). Participants will also be involved in trialing the developed smartwatch application. Similar methods (i.e. group discussion and drawings) and data analysis will be applied in each workshop.

Individuals with ASD have a range of cognitive and physical challenges, many of the lessons learned from this research could be applied to other populations with similar disabilities.

References

1. Kanner, L.: Autistic disturbances of affective contact. Nerv. Child **2**, 217–253 (1943)
2. Asperger, H.: Die "Autistischen" Psychopathen im Kindesalter. Archiv für Psychiatrie und Nervenkrankheiten **117**(1), 76–136 (1944)
3. Duncan, A.W., Bishop, S.L.: Understanding the gap between cognitive abilities and daily living skills in adolescents with autism spectrum disorders with average intelligence. Autism **19**(1), 64–72 (2015)
4. Odom, S.L., et al.: Technology-aided interventions and instruction for adolescents with autism spectrum disorder. J. Autism Dev. Disord. **45**(12), 3805–3819 (2015)
5. Frauenberger, C., Good, J., Keay-Bright, W.: Designing technology for children with special needs: bridging perspectives through participatory design. CoDesign **7**(1), 1–28 (2011)
6. Australian Bureau of Statistics. Disability, Ageing and carers, Australia: summary of findings, 2015. Australian Bureau of Statistics. Commonwealth of Australia, Canberra (2015). http://www.abs.gov.au/ausstats/abs@.nsf/mf/4430.0. Accessed 3 Mar 2018
7. Hourcade, J.P., Bullock-Rest, N.E., Hansen, T.E.: Multitouch tablet applications and activities to enhance the social skills of children with autism spectrum disorders. Pers. Ubiquitous Comput. J. Article **16**(2), 157–168 (2012)
8. Kuo, M.H., Orsmond, G.I., Coster, W.J., Cohn, E.S.: Media use among adolescents with autism spectrum disorder. Autism **18**(8), 914–923 (2014)
9. Mazurek, M.O., Shattuck, P.T., Wagner, M., Cooper, B.P.: Prevalence and correlates of screen-based media use among youths with autism spectrum disorders. J. Autism Dev. Disord. **42**(8), 1757–1767 (2012)
10. Phillips, B., Zhao, H.: Predictors of assistive technology abandonment. Assist. Technol. **5**(1), 36–45 (1993)
11. King, A.M., Thomeczek, M., Voreis, G., Scott, V.: iPad® use in children and young adults with Autism Spectrum Disorder: an observational study. Child Lang. Teach. Ther. **30**(2), 159–173 (2014)
12. Nielsen, J.: Usability Engineering, 1st edn. Morgan Kaufmann, Elsevier, New York (1994)
13. Scherer, M.J.: Assistive Technology: Matching Device and Consumer for Successful Rehabilitation. American Psychological Association, Worcester (2002)
14. Norman, D.: The Design of Everyday Things: Revised and Expanded Edition. Basic Books, New York City (2013)
15. Fuad-Luke, A.: Design Activism: Beautiful Strangeness for a Sustainable World. Routledge, London (2013)

16. Norman, D.A.: Human-centered design considered harmful. Interactions **12**(4), 14–19 (2005)
17. Frauenberger, C., Good, J., Alcorn, A.: Challenges, opportunities and future perspectives in including children with disabilities in the design of interactive technology. In: Proceedings of the 11th International Conference on Interaction Design and Children, pp. 367–370. ACM (2012)
18. Francis, P., Balbo, S., Firth, L.: Towards co-design with users who have autism spectrum disorders. Univ. Access Inf. Soc. **8**(3), 123–135 (2009)
19. Madsen, M., El Kaliouby, R., Eckhardt, M., Hoque, M.E., Goodwin, M.S., Picard, R.: Lessons from participatory design with adolescents on the autism spectrum. In: Extended Abstracts on Human Factors in Computing Systems, CHI 2009, pp. 3835–3840, ACM, Boston (2009)
20. Malinverni, L., Mora-Guiard, J., Padillo, V., Mairena, M., Hervás, A., Pares, N.: Participatory design strategies to enhance the creative contribution of children with special needs. In: Proceedings of the 2014 Conference on Interaction Design and Children, IDC 2014, pp. 85–94, ACM, Aarhus (2014)
21. Madden, D., Cadet-James, Y., Atkinson, I., Watkin Lui, F.: Probes and prototypes: a participatory action research approach to codesign. CoDesign **10**(1), 31–45 (2014)

Data Fusion Network for Instance Segmentation

Lifu Wang, Weinan Li, and Yan Kang[⊠]

Sino-Dutch Biomedical and Information Engineering School,
Northeastern University, Shenyang 110169, China
wanglifu@stumail.neu.edu.cn, kangy@neusoft.com

Abstract. We propose a Mask-Ensemble method for instance segmentation of cell nucleus. We are primarily motivated by the need of developmental biology to quantify the cell nucleus, which can help medical experts with image diagnosis. A new image segmentation algorithm of nucleus is proposed based on convolutional neural networks which combines with data augmentation strategies. First, the classified nucleus are used to train fusion layer parameters. Next, the image augmentation strategy is used to expand the original image to eight inputs, and the image color contrast is improved. At the end, the best ensemble strategy for each type of nucleus is trained for prediction. The proposed algorithm effectively reduces the redundancy of image local information and obtains the boundary position of the target area more accurately.

Keywords: Deep learning · Instance segmentation
Data augmentation strategy · Cell nucleus segmentation

1 Introduction

The research for automatic analysis of microscopy images depends on robust cell nucleus segmentation. This is the basis for understanding cell functions, tissue development and disease progression. Due to the numerous cell nucleus, cell segmentation is a complicated and huge task, which cannot only rely on human visual recognition. Solving such cell detection problems by computer is ideal and practical. However, it is quite challenging because of poor staining, variable fluorescence in cells or cell organelles, low contrast, high nucleus density, deformable nucleus shapes and appearance variation, etc. [1, 2]. All of these factors affect the accuracy of the segmentation algorithm, resulting in the error of segmentation results. Therefore, it is important to obtain a robust and reliable segmentation of nucleus via automatic methods.

Several segmentation methods for cell nucleus segmentation have been proposed based on traditional image processing algorithms including region growing, thresholding morphological operations and watershed [3]. However, a few limitations are reported in the previous work: (i) The traditional image separation methods are usually not effective and are only applicable to certain imaging modes. (e.g. optical image instead of electron microscopy) (ii) Previous methods are not fully automatic as they

S. Siuly et al. (Eds.): HIS 2018, LNCS 11148, pp. 175–182, 2018.
https://doi.org/10.1007/978-3-030-01078-2_16

typically require either pre-processing, hand-selected features for cells and/or post-processing.

In recent research, deep learning methods have become a widely used and accepted methods in the field of computer vision. Convolutional neural networks (CNNs) are particularly suited to image classification [4–6] and semantic segmentation [7]. Cell nucleus segmentation is one of the popular applications of CNNs. The Mask R-CNN [8] architecture introduced by He has inspired many segmentation applications. Based on Fast/Faster R-CNN [9, 10], a fully convolutional network (FCN) is applied to mask prediction, along with box regression and classification. To achieve high performance, feature pyramid network (FPN) is utilized to extract in-network feature hierarchy, where a top-down path with lateral connections is augmented to propagate semantically strong features.

In this paper, we present a data ensemble method for microscopy cell nucleus images, which achieves better performance than the existing cell nucleus segmentation methods on datasets from Kaggle 2018 Data Science Bowl. Our main contributions are as follows: (i) By expanding the original Mask R-CNN network, we improved the accuracy of the individual cell nucleus segmentation masks. We predict the final individual nucleus mask by extending one image to eight, which reduces errors from lighting, blurry borders and overlapping. (ii) The best ensemble parameters are trained to classify different types of cell nucleus, such as nerve cells and blood cells.

2 Methods

2.1 Data Expansion

The proposed network requires boundary boxes for training, but generally available ground truth data has very few cell nucleus with boundary boxes. This limited training data is insufficient to allow the model to learn the invariance required in nucleus appearance and shape variation. Illumination has a great influence on the semantic segmentation of pixels. We can enhance the brightness and contrast of the input images by adjusting gamma value, which makes it easier to distinguish the image details when the gray value is low. Unlike natural objects, the nucleus in a microscopic image can be presented in any orientation, so we use warping and geometrical transformations (rotations, random crops, mirroring, and padding) to further increase training data.

2.2 Network Structure

The proposed cell nucleus proposal network (NPN) uses two parallel fully connected layers to predict the center anchor of the boundary boxes proposals for cell nucleus and their scores - probability being nucleus or background. It consists of two parts. The first part of the network extracts 256-dimensional feature vectors from 28×28 rectangular regions in the input images [11]. In the second part, we set up the positive and negative sample selection rules for training. If the corresponding reference box of the anchor with the ground truth IOU is greater than 0.7, the positive sample is marked. If the corresponding reference box of the anchor with the ground truth IOU is less than 0.3, the negative sample is marked (Fig. 1).

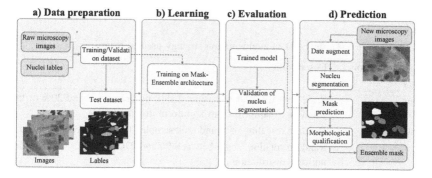

Fig. 1. Illustration of our framework

NPN uses k (=9) anchors at each pixel to propose nucleus at multiple scales and aspect ratio. Anchors can be understood as anchor points, located at the center of the n*n sliding window. In a sliding window, we can simultaneously predict multiple proposals. NPN uses 3 kinds of scales and 3 aspect ratio determining that the current sliding window corresponding to the reference boxes. The outputs of bbox layer, are the center position coordinate of reference boxes x_a, y_a and width height w_a, h_a. [12]

$$b_i = \left(\frac{x - x_a}{w_a}, \frac{y - y_a}{h_a}, \log\left(\frac{w}{w_a}\right), \log\left(\frac{h}{h_a}\right)\right) \tag{1}$$

The architecture is inspired by the original Mask R-CNN model. We introduce the "Data ensemble layer" at the back of the network. It consists of two steps. First we classify the nucleus of the Mask R-CNN network training dataset and train the network until the loss function converges. This is when the trained model will have a preliminary recognition and segmentation effect on the nucleus. Then we set the model trained in the first step to "test mode" and start training backend fusion network. We support a variety of fusion strategies: majority vote, averaging, use raw probability scores or threshold labels. (i) We consider the bounding box of each mask. We merge the boxes (new bounding box encloses all overlapping boxes) and sum the masks if the overlap in bounding boxes between masks is more than threshold. (ii) Select masks based on a voting threshold e.g. if more than 50% of cases designated a pixel as 1, then assign 1 to that pixel. (iii) Average the semantic mask output and select pixels based on a voting threshold. During the training, we expand each image to 8 images, and the 8 data enhanced images are input into the whole network as a batch. A data augmentation strategy is used on the input patches in order to reduce over fitting and improve generalization [6, 13, 14]. The strategy includes random shifting, rotation, rescaling, flipping and blurring. Table 1 summarizes the most common data augmentation methods and the corresponding parameters we adjust. The seven augment methods in Table 1 are all used for input images (augment2, augment3…augment8) of Fig. 2. The inputs of data ensemble layer are the batch's prediction results (nuclear Mask area and cell type) based on the Mask R-CNN network. In the final, the fusion layer parameters are optimized and the optimal fusion strategies of different types of nucleus are obtained through training.

Table 1. Data augmentation strategy used in fusion

Data augmentation strategy	Description
Shifting	Random horizontal and vertical shifting between 0 and 20% of the patch size, sampled from a uniform distribution
Rescaling	Random rescaling of a randomly sampled factor between 1/0.8 and 1.2
Rotation	Random rotation, angle between 90 and 270 degrees, sampled from a uniform distribution
Flipping 1	Random flipping: vertical flipping
Flipping 2	Random flipping: horizontal flipping
Blurring	Random blurring: Gaussian blur with the standard deviation of the Gaussian kernel being uniformly sampled between 0 and 4
Sharpening	Random Sharpening: Laplacian operator with Sharpened pixel being uniformly sampled between 0 and 5

3 Training

In the training phase, the model is trained 18 k iterations at the learning rate of 0.001, with the momentum changing from 0.7 to 0.9. Because it can achieve the quicker convergence results and make a few samples batch normalization, ensuring the stable training later. 8 images (1 image per GPU) are in one image batch. ResNet-50 is taken as the initial model on dataset. A dropout rate of 0.25 is used in the convolutional layers to reduce the risk of overfitting and improve generalization. The training phase takes 10 h on the NVIDIA GTX1080. Mask R-CNN outputs a binary mask for each ROI. The loss function is:

$$L = L_{cls} + L_{box} + L_{mask} \tag{2}$$

Ensemble-loss: Comparing the finally ensemble mask with Ground truth in pixel level, we obtain the following loss function:

$$L_{enloss} = \frac{\sum_1^n |P_{prediction} - P_{groundtruth}|}{\sum_1^n |P_{groundtruth}|} \tag{3}$$

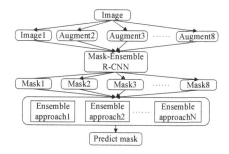

Fig. 2. Mask prediction with data ensemble layer

4 Experiments

4.1 Dataset

The proposed method is evaluated in two public available nuclei segmentation datasets. One is a multiple organ H&E stained image dataset. It consists of 30 images and the resolution of each is 1000×1000, getting from 7 organs, including the breast, liver, kidney, prostate, bladder, colon and stomach. These 30 images are split randomly into two subsets: 80% is for training, and the rest is for testing.

The second dataset comes from the Kaggle 2018 Data Science Bowl competition. This dataset contains two stages. Our models are trained on stage1_train subset for a total of 670 images and report results on the stage2_test. The stage1_train dataset contains segmentation masks for all nucleus in ground truth (GT). The challenges of this dataset are: nucleus species, numerous nucleus clusters, low contrast and blurred edges.

4.2 Results

In this paper, the most common evaluation indicators for object detection tasks include accuracy, precision, recall and f1-measure are selected. And the calculation formulas are defined by following variables.TP indicates that the sample number of cell nucleus pixel classes are divided into cell nucleus pixel classes; TN indicates that the sample number of background pixel classes are correctly classified into background pixel classes; FP indicates that the sample number of background pixels are classified into cell nucleus pixels; FN indicates that the sample number of cell nucleus pixel classes are divided into background pixel classes.

In order to evaluate the effectiveness of the proposed algorithm, a number of common image segmentation methods and the original Mask R-CNN model methods are selected as the comparison algorithms, and the results are compared with our algorithm. WATERSHED is a morphological image segmentation method based on topological theory. FCM is a segmentation algorithm based on fuzzy theory, which uses membership degree to determine each pixel point of an image belongs to each category. SegNet [15] uses decoders to sample up low resolution input feature maps. In addition, U-Net [16] end-to-end network is also used as the comparison algorithm. The results of the operation on each algorithm are shown in Table 2. The comparison of cell nucleus image segmentation results of algorithms are shown in Fig. 3.

Table 2. Comparison of each cell nucleus segmentation algorithm

Method	Accuracy (%)	Precision (%)	Recall (%)	F1-measure (%)
WATERSHED	83.62	60.77	87.45	71.71
FCM	85.34	67.52	91.49	77.70
SegNet	89.48	68.76	93.49	79.24
U-Net	90.21	77.90	87.31	82.34
Mask R-CNN	91.03	83.41	83.46	83.44
Mask-ensemble R-CNN	93.72	88.58	82.62	85.50

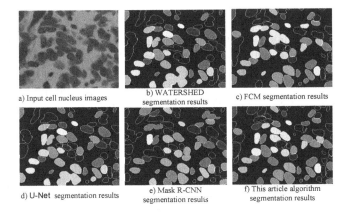

a) Input cell nucleus images   b) WATERSHED segmentation results   c) FCM segmentation results

d) U-Net segmentation results   e) Mask R-CNN segmentation results   f) This article algorithm segmentation results

Fig. 3. Comparison of segmentation results of each algorithm

As shown in Table 2, the algorithm proposed in this paper is superior to the other contrast algorithms on the three evaluation indexes of accuracy, precision and recall. We note that if there are multiple overlap from different augmentations, the prediction is confident and mostly correct. The color variety is well controlled by the ensemble procedure on test augmentation. Figure 4 shows a visual comparison between our method and original Mask R-CNN. As shown in the sample image, we can find that the segmentation error on the first image is mainly caused by under-segmentation and missing detections. While our segmentation result has fewer false negatives and higher accuracy in terms of nuclei boundaries than original Mask R-CNN.

We do not need perfect labels to learn but we do need many labels per sample if they are ambiguous. This is why pseudo-labels from ensemble classifiers should work. The distilling knowledge from ensemble is shown in Fig. 5.

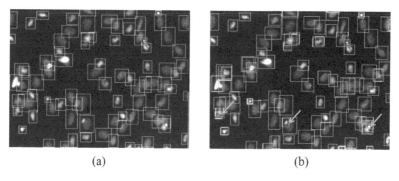

Fig. 4. Comparison of the results (a) Mask R-CNN (b) proposed method

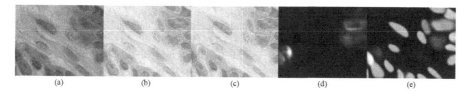

Fig. 5. (a) example of original histopathology images (b, c) corresponding images after augmentation (d) masks ensemble (e) final segmentation results

5 Conclusion

In this paper, we have presented a Mask-Ensemble method, which performs cell nucleus segmentation by "Data ensemble layer" at the back of the network. Experiments demonstrated that our data augmentation strategy for ensemble method performs better on a challenging dataset compared to other similar current cell nucleus segmentation methods. In future work, we will explore learning procedures that adapt weights in the critical contour regions to improve the accuracy of the results by training more data.

Acknowledgments. I am highly thankful for the support and guidance from Sino-Dutch Biomedical and Information Engineering School, Northeastern University, Shenyang, China.

References

1. Buggenthin, F., Marr, C., Schwarzfischer, M., et al.: An automatic method for robust and fast cell detection in bright field images from high-throughput microscopy. BMC Bioinform. **14** (1), 200–203 (2013)
2. Metin, N.G., Laura, B., Ali, C., Anant, M., Nasir, R., Bulent, Y.: Histopathological image analysis: a review. IEEE Rev. Biomed. Eng. **2**, 147–171 (2008)

3. Adollah, R., Mashor, M.Y., Nasir, N.F.M., et al.: Blood cell image segmentation: a review. In: Abu Osman, N.A., Ibrahim, F., Wan Abas, W.A.B., Abdul Rahman, H.S., Ting, H.N. (eds.) 4th Kuala Lumpur International Conference on Biomedical Engineering, vol. 21, pp. 141–144. Springer, Heidelberg (2008). https://doi.org/10.1007/978-3-540-69139-6_39

4. Ciresan, D.C., Meier, U., Gambardella, L.M., Schmidhuber, J.: Convolutional neural network committees for handwritten character classification. In: 2011 International Conference on Document Analysis and Recognition, pp. 1135–1139 (2011)

5. Karpathy, A., Toderici, G., Shetty, S., Leung, T.: Large-scale video classification with convolutional neural networks. In: Proceedings of the (2014)

6. Simonyan, K., Zisserman, A.: Very deep convolutional networks for large-scale image recognition. arXiv [cs.CV] (2014)

7. Long, J., Shelhamer, E., Darrell, T.: Fully convolutional networks for semantic segmentation. In: Proceedings IEEE (2015)

8. He, K., Gkioxari, G., Dollár, P., Girshick, R.B.: Mask R-CNN. In: ICCV (2017)

9. Girshick, R.: Fast R-CNN. In: Ren, S., He, K., Girshick, R., Sun, J. (eds.) ICCV (2015)

10. Faster R-CNN: Towards real-time object detection with region proposal networks. In: NIPS (2015)

11. Zeiler, M.D., Fergus, R.: Visualizing and understanding convolutional networks. In: European Conference on Computer Vision (ECCV) (2014)

12. Ren, S., He, K., Girshick, R., Sun, J.: Faster R-CNN: towards real-time object detection with region proposal networks. In: Advances in Neural Information Processing Systems (NIPS) (2015)

13. Krizhevsky, A., Sutskever, I., Hinton, G.E.: ImageNet classification with deep convolutional neural networks. In: Advances in Neural Information Processing Systems 25 (NIPS) (2012)

14. Pereira, F., Burges, C.J.C., Bottou, L., Weinberger, K.Q.: Processing Systems. Neural Information, vol. 25, pp. 1097–1105. Curran Associates, Inc., Red Hook (2012)

15. Badrinarayanan, V., Kendall, A., Cipolla, R.: SegNet: a deep convolutional encoder-decoder architecture for image segmentation. In: Computer Vision and Pattern Recognition (cs.CV) (2015)

16. Ronneberger, O., Fischer, P., Brox, T.: U-Net: convolutional networks for biomedical image segmentation. In: Navab, N., Hornegger, J., Wells, W.M., Frangi, A.F. (eds.) MICCAI 2015. LNCS, vol. 9351, pp. 234–241. Springer, Cham (2015). https://doi.org/10.1007/978-3-319-24574-4_28

Intensity Thinking as a Shared Challenge in Consumer-Targeted eHealth

Marjo Rissanen[(✉)]

Aalto University School of Science, Espoo, Finland
mkrissan@gmail.com

Abstract. There is high production intensity in eHealth, and it is therefore recognized that models and methods are also needed when trying to develop customer-centered applications and systems. The purpose of translational medicine is to offer high-quality services, better health outcomes, and efficiency through innovations. The aim of this analysis is to clarify the importance of intensity thinking in the eHealth sector as a common design challenge of professionals and cooperators. Awareness of intensity thinking is one key area of consideration when reaching for translational design targets in eHealth, and it is thus also useful in the diagnostic and formative evaluation phases. Cooperation by different professionals is needed when creating common aims and missions in eHealth design. When aspects of care intensity are comprehended as fundamental to evaluation strategies, a more solid basis for successful innovation policy can be reached.

Keywords: Intensity thinking · Quality · Translational design
eHealth evaluation

1 Introduction

Consideration of care intensity is a meaningful issue in eHealth design and production. Health-consumer-targeted translational eHealth design aspires to successful health outcomes, better levels of health. eHealth interventions promote patient engagement and enhance clinical outcomes [1]. On the other hand, there is also confusion among health professionals and health consumers about e.g., which mHealth products are reliable and rely on evidence-based medicine [2]. Consumer-targeted eHealth serves its main purpose in health care as a process supporter in health management (preventive, curative, and follow-up processes), information and knowledge enhancement, and interaction assistance between health service users and professionals. Intensity thinking in health care focuses on investigating questions of appropriate and reasonable resource use and quality of care, such as whether resource inputs are adequate in professional health care practices. As such, intensity thinking is intertwined with versatile quality thinking. In eHealth, the question is how to innovatively enhance the intensity of care processes. This type of thinking considers economic consequences, but it is especially concerned with high-quality services. The purpose of the health sector is to offer services that reflect high professionalism and high-quality clinical outcomes.

© Springer Nature Switzerland AG 2018
S. Siuly et al. (Eds.): HIS 2018, LNCS 11148, pp. 183–192, 2018.
https://doi.org/10.1007/978-3-030-01078-2_17

Methods and tools are needed to facilitate translational processes in health care [3]. Translational research aims to assess implementation of standards, effectiveness, efficiency, quality, and outcomes of care [4] and reorganizes and coordinates systems of care [5]. Although a challenge to achieve [6], cooperation between eHealth designers, health professionals, and other cooperators is underlined in translational eHealth informatics as a requirement for better synergy [7]. Production intensity in eHealth is high, meaning that deeper concentration on knowledge bases and theory frames is important. Awareness and comprehension of intensity challenges in care helps eHealth designers and cooperators better reach translational design targets [8]. The aim of this position analysis is to clarify this shared design challenge.

2   Intensity as Part of Knowledge Frames of Design

In this analysis, care intensity thinking is considered a knowledge factor that should have a position in the theoretical framing of eHealth design. It represents theoretical understanding, which helps streamline eHealth design practices. Its comprehension enhances synergy between practice and theory, which is underlined in good design [9, 10]. Hevner et al. [11] divide the information systems research framework (ISRF) into the following areas: environment, IS research, and knowledge bases. In this model, a knowledge base contains foundations and methodologies that serve design and also ensure research rigor. In refinement and assessment work, all evaluative information also adds to the knowledge base. Environments consist of people, organizations, and technology that form needs and relevance for design and connected research [11].

Agarwal and Lucas [12] focus on the transformational potential and impact of information technology. Intensity evaluation in the health sector is concerned with resource use, its justification, and its impact value. Health outcomes indicate how successful intensity level input has been. Design artifacts and design theory can also have potential practical and research significance [10]. In eHealth, the practical significance of artifacts indicates the intensity value and capability of products. This significance, health outcome informs whether an artifact under evaluation can help adequately intensify health care processes (Fig. 1). Outcomes can also "be defined in terms of improvement of functional status and social participation rather" than only in terms of disease-specific outcomes [13]. Partnership with patients, health care professionals, and co-operators "can help reduce waste in the production and reporting of research evidence" [13].

Intensity consideration indicates a value mechanism that brings rigor to design practices, organizations, and technologies in eHealth. When intensity thinking is seen as one key component of knowledge bases and theory framing, behind design and evaluation, it also needs to be considered in design practice. This analysis considers how intensity thinking as a concept of design should be comprehended by IT professionals and cooperators by focusing on the following questions: (1) Why does intensity thinking need space as an evaluative tool in translational eHealth design? (2) How should designers and other groups (cooperators) in the contextual environment comprehend this theme in evaluative procedures? Key areas of intensity evaluation are

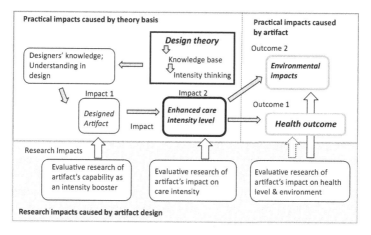

Fig. 1. DSR impacts and intensity thinking in eHealth

considered in each group at the macro level of quality. This analysis relies on literature in the contextual research field to explore this question.

3 Understanding Intensity Thinking in the Health Sector

Care intensity is a significant research area in the health sector. Broadly in clinical health practice, care intensity indicates the degree or type to which patients receive different kinds of services in their care episodes. Intensity of care has been measured according to the prevalence or type of specific service units (medical testing e.g. laboratory and radiology services, and diagnostic imaging [14], investigations, medical treatments or treatment styles [15], hospital days, health systems [16], physiotherapy [17], physical activity and exercise intensity [18], medicine recipes [19] or other sub-services etc.). The quantities, type, or style of these services provide information about care intensity levels. Communicative interaction processes with health professionals (needed knowledge and support) or patient activation and engagement levels represent also intensity factors. eHealth solutions have a great role and potential in this challenge [1]. Professional intensity level of care can be high or low depending on the contextual requirements and it means such a level of intensity necessary to reach an adequate clinical outcome (e.g. a correct diagnosis and relevant care).

Low-level care intensity describes a situation in which the intensity or quantity of service components is low but patients still receive correct diagnoses and optimal care. Low-level care intensity is typical in situations in which a patient's problem is unambiguous and the need for care procedures, knowledge, and interactive support is minimal. Low-level care intensity is justified in these situations because declaring a patient's situation and providing a correct diagnosis and relevant care is sufficient. Low-level care intensity thus represents a professional-intensity level of care.

However, non-justified low-level care intensity describes a situation in which the intensity of clinical care or service components is too low to provide a correct diagnosis or optimal care, or in which a patient does not receive necessary knowledge or support. Non-justified low-level care intensity may lead to de-medicalization, may increase indirect costs, and it does not represent professional-level care intensity. Similarly, high-level care intensity is justified if it is needed to declare a patient's situation and guarantee high-quality care processes. In high-level care intensity, the number of service components or clinical procedures in a care process is high or intensive, as is the knowledge or support needed by patients. High-level care intensity represents professional-level care intensity. However, non-justified high-level care intensity describes a situation in which a patient is provided too much service components, treatments, care procedures etc. in relation to one's problem, without sufficient medical reason. Non-justified high-level care intensity does not represent professional-level care intensity, and it may cause unnecessary costs and increased medicalization of health care. There are different levels of analysis in medicalization–demedicalization scheme [20] like discourses (biomedical models, definitions etc.), practices (biomedical practices and technologies), and identifiers (physicians, hospitals, individual and collective actors). It is mentioned also macro (legislative), meso (mission statements), and micro levels (face-to-face-interaction, client self-management) [20, 21]. It is remarked that conceptualizations easily "understate the prevalence of demedicalization" [20]. Correspondingly care intensity issues can be considered in all these levels. Because of the complexity and nuances of medicalization-demedicalization phenomena it is also warned about over-simplistic generalizations [22]. It is also remarked that doctors can supply "assistance and support even in the absence of unequivocal diagnosis and proven therapeutic interventions" [23]. Intensity considerations in connection with their justification analysis describe the quality and efficiency of care.

Recent evidence shows that higher-intensity care often means better outcomes [17, 18, 24] or lower mortality [25], and "purely cost-focused health reform may be insufficient to achieve efficiency in healthcare delivery" [14]. The increasing prevalence of health systems and hospital-managed care may lead to higher care quality but are unlikely to reduce hospital discharge costs [16]. Higher service intensity does not always guarantee higher quality of care [26].

Consumer-targeted eHealth applications concentrate specifically on the informative and interaction areas of care intensity, but they also have a significant role as supporters of care processes in different phases (prevention, curative, and follow-up processes). Interaction between health consumers and health professionals is now generally seen as an equal communicative process in which both parties participate according to their roles. eHealth systems thus also have an important role in intensity evaluation. One objective of health-consumer-targeted eHealth is to enhance patient activation levels, and increased activation levels have been linked with better health outcomes [1]. Lower intensity in access and use of consumer-targeted eHealth systems can come from poor system availability and usability [27, 28], or from interface issues such as content that is difficult to read [28]. In particular, elderly people often lack enough support to use online services [29].

eHealth systems and applications also may represent less-than-optimal intensity levels in relation to actual needs. Here, intensity in eHealth is considered a product's ability to function as a process intensifier in its intended role and task. Products' fulfillment of this role is not necessarily dependent on the intensity requirements of design, production, and implementation. The complicacy rates of a system may mean even more challenges to its proper functioning and intensity value. Intense complicacy rates may translate to excessive time and resource requirements for users. Applications containing too many unnecessary options or activation tasks without medical justification provide little process intensification value. An application represents also too-low intensity if it is too one-sided or superficial in its intended role. Care-intensity tasks are critical, especially in situations surrounding a product that requires the re-engineering of current processes or in which human resources are substituted with artificial intelligence. Evaluative and maturation procedures are typically needed when trying to attain professional-level care intensity in eHealth.

4 Integrating Intensity Thinking with eHealth Design and Evaluation by People in Focus

4.1 Designers and Producers

Designers cooperate often with their focus environments and customers, so tasks of intensity should include common interests. Designers' attention should be focused on intensity tasks already at the very early stages of design; intensity thinking is useful in the diagnostic and formative evaluation phases and might prevent producing and designing systems that are too complex (and therefore less usable) or that lack real impact value. For practical reasons, designers' interests are typically focused on the artifact and its competence in the process. Product maturation, however, means that evaluation will continue in the later phases of impact evaluation and gathered outcome evaluation. Cooperation with focus environments makes this kind of evaluation possible.

Intensity tasks are connected with many areas of quality. *Mission-related questions* consider also targeting and ethics. Are target groups well-selected and defined? Which strategies are needed for groups or areas in which care process intensity is generally recognized as too low or in which target groups are unattainable? Creative insights have a distinct place in new artifact and design knowledge [10], and such an approach is needed to discover neglected areas of intensity.

When considering issues of *product quality and process quality*, design questions of intensity must consider design strategies and usability tasks. Is any supplementary product capable enough for its purpose or is there a need to re-engineer the processes in intensity enhancement challenges? IT systems in the health sector still tend to reinforce old models rather than create new ones [27]. Is the product based on best medical practices [2]? The complexity of an artifact is a natural focus of analytical evaluation of IT systems [11], and it is also a task that is highly connected with an artifact's intensity value. Is the product workable and fit for use with a certain engagement degree that is suitable for different focus or interest groups? Is the product streamlined enough in the eHealth sector so that its use does not require too much guidance or introduction [30, 31]? Is the product a natural part of the process in a way that does not require too much devotion to the application and its characteristics? Is functioning self-evident? Does the product adequately intensify the process in question? What patient activation level is reasonable and when are intensity levels deemed to be optimal? When considering *customer quality*, the following questions are vital: Are users' opinions considered in different stages of the design process and are designers aware of this input in the idea phase? Are there signs that the system or application is perceived as too superficial or too general (signs of a too-low intensity value)? (see Table 1, section Designer) Are there customer concerns about the system being too complex or labor-intensive, which may decrease the intensity of its use? What kind of maturation policy is planned to enhance problem areas (*quality of production*)?

Table 1. Key areas in intensity evaluation in roles

Role	Category	Key areas of evaluation
Designers	Mission	High-quality care and outcomes; optimal intensity level
	Ethics	Ethical acceptability of products
	Efficiency	Reasonable input-output ratio
	Product	Products as care intensifiers
		Evaluation of optimal intensity levels
	Process	Products as process intensifiers
		System coordination
	Production	Policy and strategy support for intensity enhancement
	Customer	Consideration of customer input; usability and complexity
	Image	Information quality
Management	Mission	High-quality care and outcomes; optimal intensity level
	Ethics	Ethical acceptability of products
		Priority thinking in balance with investments
	Efficiency	Reasonable input-output ratio
	Product	Professional expertise evaluation of utility value
		Products as care intensifiers
	Process	Products as process intensifiers
		System coordination
	Production	Policy and strategy evaluation
	Customer	Consideration of customer input
	Image	Trustworthiness evaluation of image

4.2   Management and Health Professionals

Co-design processes in design and evaluation are valuable practices, especially when trying to create new models in health care [27]. Many process intensifiers enhance the coordination and interaction between interest groups in health care processes. For these reasons, multi-professional teams are needed to evaluate tasks that deal with items of care intensity in interaction processes.

Health professionals who evaluate products' or systems' capabilities as part of health care processes are primary evaluators of tasks of *product and process quality* from the view of practice in certain medical disciplines. It is recommended that physicians should evaluate e.g., the value of consumer targeted mHealth apps because most apps have been produced without medical expert involvement [32]. Intensity optimization becomes relevant despite the intended role of certain process supporters. An important question is whether the system is competent enough to enhance care intensity levels and outcomes in its intended task. Are all functions medically meaningful? Does the system adapt flexibly to certain established processes or is it able to re-engineer processes meaningfully? Special attention to customer quality issues is also needed when evaluating user load in practice; a too-heavy load for users and professionals means lost time, does not necessarily enhance the intensity of processes, and may even mean slower processes without any added quality value. *Ethical considerations* are necessary if priority thinking is in balance with investments and when estimating reasonable input-output ratios. Are so-called urgent priority areas where care intensity should be enhanced noticed in the development of strategies and mission plans? *Images of artifacts* affect adoption decisions [33], and image issues thus represent an essential evaluation point. Are images or promises of deeper intensity values for certain products based on facts and evidence of their proper function? What kinds of maturation procedures are needed to enhance the intensity values of artifacts? (see Table 1, Management)

4.3   Health Service Users

Health service users are the focus group when assessing outcomes of care. Their role as evaluators is currently more prominent in the design process than it was previously. User experiences and flexible open channels for user feedback are necessary for efficient intensity evaluation. Designers often overestimate users' capacity and interest to engage with new procedures and tools. Users are the right people to assess suitable time and work loads that new innovations, such as self-health-management, require. They also have a role in evaluating the perceived advantages of products, as well their ethical acceptance. However, some products might increase customer satisfaction or activity levels in health management but may not be necessary or competent enough in the sense of health optimization. Therefore, the opinions of health professionals also need to be heard when the real benefits of products in health maintenance or enhancement are evaluated.

5   Discussion

Automation and technology innovations have an essential position when striving for efficient, high-quality health care [34]. Intensity thinking forms one meaningful part of the knowledge base that supports eHealth design [8]. In intensity evaluation, the following key points are important to consider:

1. What are the intended main roles of the planned artifact (preventive, curative, or follow-up procedures, knowledge- and information sharing, support of interactions)?
2. How does the artifact enhance care intensity levels?
3. Is there an area in which the intensity level is recognized as being too low?
4. Is the application capable of intensifying processes in a way that will satisfy all parties? What kinds of maturation procedures are needed?
5. Are there blind spots in the protocol in which intensity tasks are neglected? How are they being dealt with?
6. Are supplementary products competent or is it necessary to re-engineer the processes in intensity enhancement challenges?
7. Is intensity policy observed for products that represent artificial intelligence?

If intensity issues are understood as a broader concept with connection to several quality aspects instead of as a resource question, their operationalization means more concrete tasks for different professionals. The rapid growth of health consumer targeted eHealth requires that evaluation of the justification of intensity levels is necessary. An essential question is whether investments, components, and changes in IT structure produce remarkable enhancements in intensity tasks and if the acquired intensity level of care represents high-quality care.

It is understandable that eHealth may produce both efficiency and cost savings if human resources, the most significant cost factor in the health sector, can be replaced by applications such as artificial intelligence or robotics. Intensity evaluation is necessary to move forward and replace humans with IT products or services without damaging professional-level care intensity. This issue is about the unintended consequences of IT [35] if savings happen at the expense of quality. Targeting optimal intensity levels in health care is a common aim for which the cooperation of different interest groups is needed. Synergy of different views in intensity tasks is useful in translational design aspirations. Co-design processes in this area, however, have their challenges; "health professionals and users may easily focus on old and well-known problems and solutions, and novel innovations by IT designers may remain untapped if users' needs are not addressed" [36]. The success of a design research project requires research, cognitive (creativity, reasoning), and social skills in designing innovative solutions and in bringing together collective knowledge [37].

Intensity thinking and its justification analysis represent evaluation that is closely connected to all other quality aspects, and it highlights management informed by results and efficient resource use, along with overall quality. Evaluation in eHealth is not straightforward, so innovative models and strategies are needed to support reasoned design. This means that intensity issues connect also macro (legislative) and meso (mission) levels of evaluation. Intensity thinking as part of the current foundation of innovation policy in eHealth requires more attention and design strategies that consider these fundamental issues. Priority challenges mean that intensity levels must be increased for the right tasks and actions.

References

1. Barello, S., Triberti, S., Graffigna, G., Libreri, C., Serino, S., Hibbard, J., Riva, G.: eHealthfor patient engagement: a systematic review. Front. Psychol. **6**, 1–13 (2016)
2. Larson, R.: A path to better-quality mHealth apps. JMIR Mhealth Uhealth **6**(7), 10414 (2018). https://doi.org/10.2196/10414
3. Wehling, M.: Translational medicine science or wishful thinking? J. Transl. Med. **6**(1), 1–3 (2008)
4. Narayan, K.V., Benjamin, E., Gregg, E.W., Norris, S.L., Engelgau, M.M.: Diabetes translation research: where are we and where do we want to be? Ann. Intern. Med. **140**(11), 958–963 (2004)
5. Woolf, S.: The meaning of translational research and why it matters. JAMA **299**(2), 211–213 (2008)
6. Sarkar, I.: Biomedical informatics and translational medicine. J. Transl. Med. **8**, 22 (2010)
7. Polese, F., Capunzo, M.: The determinants of translational medicine success: a managerial contribution. Transl. Med. @ UniSa **6**, 29 (2013)
8. Rissanen, M.: Integrating translational design ideology for consumer-targeted, informative eHealth. Int. J. Innov. Manag. Technol. **7**(6), 260–265 (2016)
9. Hevner, A.: A three cycle view of design science research. Scand. J. Inf. Syst. **19**(2), 87–92 (2007)
10. Baskerville, R., Baiyere, A., Gregor, S., Hevner, A., Rossi, M.: Design science research contributions: finding a balance between artifact and theory. J. Assoc. Inf. Syst. **19**(5), 358–376 (2018)
11. Hevner, A., March, S., Park, J.: Design science information system research. MIS Q. **26**(1), 75–105 (2004)
12. Agarwal, R., Lucas Jr., H.C.: The information systems identity crisis: focusing on high-visibility and high-impact research. MIS Q. **29**(3), 381–398 (2005)
13. Royen, P., Rees, C., Groenewegen, E.: Patient-centred interprofessional collaboration in primary care: Challenges for clinical, educational, and health services research. An EGPRN Keynote paper. Eur. J. Gen. Pract. **20**, 327–332 (2014)
14. Abaluck, J., Agha, L., Kabrhel, C., Raja, A., Venkatesh, A.: The determinants of productivity in medical testing: intensity and allocation of care. Am. Econ. Rev. **106**(12), 3730–3764 (2016)
15. Silber, J.H., Kaestner, R., Even-Shoshan, O., Wang, Y., Bressler, L.J.: Aggressive treatment style and surgical outcomes. Health Serv. Res. **45**(6p2), 1872–1892 (2010)
16. Henke, R.M., et al.: Impact of health system affiliation on hospital resource use intensity and quality of care. Health Serv. Res. **53**(1), 63–86 (2018)
17. Taylor, N.: High-intensity acute hospital physiotherapy for patients with hip fracture may improve functional independence and can reduce hospital length of stay. J. Physiother. **63**(1), 50 (2017)
18. Hsu, B., Merom, D., Blyth, F., Naganathan, V., Handelsman, D., Cumming, R.: Temporal relationship between physical activity exercise intensity, and mortality in older men. Innov. Aging **1**(suppl 1), 1052 (2017)
19. Hylek, E.M., et al.: Effect of intensity of oral anticoagulation on stroke severity and mortality in atrial fibrillation. N. Engl. J. Med. **349**(11), 1019–1026 (2003)
20. Halfmann, D.: Recognizing medicalisation and demedicalisation: discourses, practices, and identities. Health **16**(2), 186–207 (2011)
21. Scambler, G., Britten, M.: System, lifeworld and doctor-patient interaction. In: Scambler, G. (ed.) Habermas, Critical Theory and Health, pp. 45–67. Routledge, London (2001)

22. Lowenberg, J., Davis, F.: Beyond medicalisation-demedicalisation: the case of holistic health. Sociol. Health Illn. **16**(5), 579–599 (1994)
23. Broom, D.H., Woodward, R.V.: Medicalisation reconsidered: toward a collaborative approach to care. Sociol. Health Illn. **18**(3), 357–378 (1996)
24. Burke, L., Ryan, A.: The complex relationship between cost and quality in US healthcare. Virtual Mentor Am. Med. Assoc. J. Ethics **2**, 124–130 (2014)
25. Lerolle, N., Trinquart, L., Bornstain, C., Tadié, J.M., Imbert, A., Diehl, J.L., et al.: Increased intensity of treatment and decreased mortality in elderly patients in an intensive care unit over a decade. Crit. Care Med. **38**(1), 59–64 (2010)
26. Friesner, D., Rosenman, R.: The relationship between service intensity and the quality of health care: an exploratory data analysis. Health Serv. Manag. Res. **18**(1), 41–52 (2005)
27. Øvretveit, J.: Digital technologies supporting person-centered integrated care: a perspective. Int. J. Integr. Care **17**(4), 1–4 (2017). https://doi.org/10.5334/ijic.3051
28. Kim, H., Xie, B.: Health literacy in the eHealth era: a systematic review of the literature. Patient Educ. Couns. **100**(6), 1073–1082 (2017)
29. Makai, P., Perry, M., Robben, S.H., Schers, H.J., Heinen, M.M., Rikkert, M.G.O., Melis, R. F.: Evaluation of an eHealth intervention in chronic care for frail older people: why adherence is the first target. J. Med. Internet Res. **16**(6), e156 (2014). https://doi.org/10.2196/jmir.3057
30. Rosson, M., Carroll, J.: Minimalist design for informal learning in community computing. In: Van Den Besselaar, P., De Michelis, G., Preece, J., Simone, C. (eds.) Communities and Technologies, pp. 75–94. Springer, Berlin (2005). https://doi.org/10.1007/1-4020-3591-8_5
31. Rissanen, M.: "Machine beauty"—should it inspire ehealth designers? In: Zhang, Y., Yao, G., He, J., Wang, L., Smalheiser, N.R., Yin, X. (eds.) HIS 2014. LNCS, vol. 8423, pp. 1–11. Springer, Cham (2014). https://doi.org/10.1007/978-3-319-06269-3_1
32. Cook, V.E., Ellis, A.K., Hildebrand, K.J.: Mobile health applications in clinical practice: pearls, pitfalls, and key considerations. Ann Allergy Asthma Immunol. Aug. **117**(2), 143–149 (2016)
33. Moore, G.C., Benbasat, I.: Development of an instrument to measure the perceptions of adopting an information technology innovation. Inf. Syst. Res. **2**(3), 192–222 (1991)
34. Zwicker, M., Seitz, J., Wickramasinghe, N.: Identifying critical issues for developing successful e-Health solutions. In: Wickramasinghe, N., Al-Hakim, L., Gonzalez, C., Tan, J. (eds.) Lean Thinking for Healthcare. HDIA, pp. 207–224. Springer, New York (2014). https://doi.org/10.1007/978-1-4614-8036-5_12
35. Majchrzak, A., Markus, M.L., Wareham, J.: Designing for digital transformation: lessons for information systems research from the study of ICT and societal challenges. MIS Q. **40**(2), 267–277 (2016)
36. Aidemark, J., Askenäs, L., Nygårdh, A., Strömberg, A.: User involvement in the co-design of self-care support systems for heart failure patients. Procedia Comput. Sci. **64**, 118–124 (2015)
37. Gregor, S., Hevner, A.: Positioning and presenting design science research for maximum impact. MIS Q. **37**(2), 337–355 (2013)

Web-Service Medical Messenger – Intelligent Algorithm of Remote Counseling

Nikita Shklovskiy-Kordi[1]([⊠]), Rostislav Borodin[2], Boris Zingerman[2],
Michael Shifrin[3], Olga Kremenetskaya[4], and Andrei Vorobiev[1,4]

[1] National Center for Hematology, Moscow 125167, Russia
nikitashk@gmail.com
[2] TelePat, Novoslobodskaya, 14/19, Moscow 196787, Russia
[3] Burdenko Neurosurgical Centre, Moscow 102346, Russia
[4] Center for Theoretical Problems of Physicochemical Pharmacology,
Moscow 119991, Russia

Abstract. The personal messaging channel is beneficial for the patient-doctor communication: the patient asks when the question arises and the doctor answers at the first opportunity. A PRINCIPAL ADVANTAGE over a telephone conversation is that the doctor has a convenient access to the medical history of the patient. Data preservation becomes its constructive part. The doctor's answers are supported by information templates: standard test sets, preparation for the visit, schedule and link to the site where one can make an appointment with the doctor. In this way, an effective monitoring of adherence to treatment can be realized.

Keywords: Distant medical monitoring
Medical messaging intelligent algorithms · Adherence to treatment

1 Introduction

Telemedicine Authorization began operating in Russia in 2018 [1]. Communication of the patient and the doctor has always included elements of telemedicine. The patient could write a letter or send a telegram. With the advent of phones remote counseling became almost the norm, especially after the emergence of mobile phones. Modern ICT for more than 40 years have given impetus to the development of "heavy" telemedicine with all its complex problems [2].

However, "telemedicine-light" received no less development: the patient and doctor communicate with the help of e-mail, and a little later with the help of various messengers. And it is the subject of "asymmetrical communication" that needs special Intelligent algorithm that could be generally accepted [3].

Popular messengers such as WhatsApp, Viber, Telegram, etc. are unable to solve the problems of communication between the patient and the doctor adequately: medical communication should take place in certain legal frameworks, including not only the protection of personal data and the financial information. Both the doctor and the patient should be protected from the incidents that could occur when the communication is remote [4].

© Springer Nature Switzerland AG 2018
S. Siuly et al. (Eds.): HIS 2018, LNCS 11148, pp. 193–197, 2018.
https://doi.org/10.1007/978-3-030-01078-2_18

It should be taken into account, that the communication between the patient and the doctor is asymmetric and chaotic. The initiator of communication is almost always the patient, who very often misinterprets the polite phrase of the doctor "Call me at any time." As a result the burden of doctors becomes exorbitant.

The proposed MM (Medical Messaging) project allows approaching the solution of these problems. Both the design of the project and its business model are built in such a way that they will allow the entire process of communication to be realized in certain legislative frameworks and relieve the stress – that may arise due to the asymmetry of the doctor-patient communication process [5]. We recognize this approach as Medical Messaging Intelligent Algorithm (MMIA) [6].

2   Methods

The service can be offered by medical organizations to their patients as an additional paid service,: a personal confidential communication channel is created between the patient and the doctor in a mode that is unavailable to the traditional messengers (see Fig. 1).

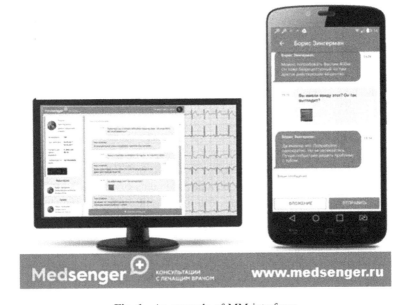

Fig. 1. An example of MM interfaces

The patient asks when the question arises, and the doctor answers whenever possible (within the time agreed in the contract, for example, 24 h). Files can also be attached to the messages.

At the request of the customer MM can be integrated with patient's EHR or PHR and telemonitoring devices. Unlike the universal messenger, the channel between the patient and the doctor is created by the administrator of the medical organization after the patient has paid under the contract and is automatically closed after the contract is terminated. In fact, it is a paid, more convenient, controlled and logged analogue of the system where doctor gives his mobile phone number or e-mail to the patient.

However, after completion of the contract, the patient does not have any personal contacts of the doctor, but all correspondence remains.

The cost of the service (price list) is determined by the medical organization independently, and also organization independently enters into a contract with the patient and charges him a fee.

Such a contract is beneficial: to the patient - he receives guaranteed support and competent help; to the doctor - the service is simple and convenient and allows responding to the patient's questions in spare time. Doctors can count on a legal remuneration for each contract they lead; the medical organization - receives additional income and acquires a competitive advantage.

Why is it Better than a Phone? The patient does not risk calling at the wrong time and distracting the doctor from an urgent matter. People usually formulate their problems in writing more clearly than in an oral conversation. The patient can attach documents, test results or photographs to specify questions. The doctor is able to understand the question and the whole complex of problems more accurately, and provide answers more fully

Technical Implementation. The service is provided to the medical organization in the form of a completely ready ("turnkey") cloud solution that does not require installation on computers or a server. For the work you need only access to the Internet. To answer questions (in particular during off-hours), doctors can also use their personal computers, tablets or telephones. Both the doctor and the patient can write messages on the computer (in the personal account) or/and in the special mobile applications (Android, iOS). In this case, all correspondence is logged and available on any device.

Service Managing. To manage the service (activation, accounting and control of contracts), the organization receives a special cloud "administrator's office". Starting the service does not require any preliminary investment. The service provider actually provides information services of communication. This service can be most in demand by:

- Patients discharged after surgery or other inpatient treatment. The new service will allow them to stay in touch with their attending physicians for the entire period of home care and rehabilitation.
- Patients with chronic disease who remain in contact with their attending physicians in the intervals between face-to-face visits.
- Parents of young children who would like to keep in touch with their pediatricians.
- Pregnant and other categories of people who are constantly monitoring their health.
- Children of elderly parents who ensure their communication with the attending physicians.
- Relatives of patients undergoing hospital treatment: the service can be offered for operative remote interaction with the attending physician, including answers to questions about the patient's condition.

Organizational and Financial Options for Patient Care. This service is not covered by state guarantees of medical care and, accordingly, can be:

- Offered as a separate paid service (a subscription for a certain period);
- included in various insurance programs;
- included in contracts for the provision of other comprehensive medical services (management of pregnancy, medical care for children or the elderly, etc.).

The medical organization concludes standard contract with the patient for the provision of paid services and accepts payment under this agreement. Together with the contract, the patient signs a special "Informed consent", including the rules and limitations of distance counseling. After that, the consultation channel between the patient and the particular physician chosen by this patient has been activated.

The organization forms the cost of services and the price list itself. The price list can include a number of services of different cost, depending on the duration, qualification or specialty of the doctor, the guaranteed speed of the doctor's response (for example, a standard contract presupposes an answer within 24 h, and in case of emergency, more expensive, within 3 h).

When determining the cost of a service, it is necessary to find a reasonable balance between the amount of money patients will be ready to pay and what additional payment doctors will be willing to receive.

It is assumed that this service will be offered by: The doctors themselves (interested in receiving additional payment). For this action, it is necessary to provide them with information materials that briefly explain the essence of the service to the patient.

The Contractual Department offers this service when contracts for other paid services are concluded. Admission Department can also offer the service during hospitalization and discharge of patients.

Information materials placed on information stands and on the web-site of a medical organization, offering "to ask your doctor in charge…" or "contact the contract department".

3   Results

48 parents of patients of the Scientific Research Institute of Emergency Children's Surgery and Traumatology of the Moscow City Health Department (ECST) were interviewed with the aid of a questionnaire. 45 of them answered that after the discharge of the child from the clinic they are ready to pay the contract price for remote consultations with the doctor who assisted this child in the clinic. The period of time that the majority of parents indicated was more than one month, 30% - about 6 months.

Three parents, who did not answer, explained that they simply did not understand what was being offered to them. In addition, many of the respondents said that they are ready to pay for such a contract not from the day of discharge but from the day the child enters the clinic.

56 doctors of ECST answered that they are ready to keep in touch with the patient for 21 days for 1000 rubles. From there, it was decided to establish the contract value in the clinic - 3000 rubles. At the same time, in order to increase further interest of the

doctors, a following decision was made - if the patient comes to make payment according to the contract on the recommendation of the doctor, 300 rubles will be paid in addition to the doctor's salary.

4 Conclusions

The proposed Medical Messaging Intelligent Algorithm can be introduced on the medicine market in Russia.

Future Development. After the adoption of the telemedicine law the number of our testers increased, especially in the state health facilities, who really need money to survive. There are still contradictions in the legislative acts. If they are eliminated, a sharp take-off is expected - percentage of moms of toddlers, pregnant women, patients during rehabilitation, chronic patients who are ready to use the service will be close to 90%. One of the latest polls showed that the entry of telemedicine into the everyday life of Russians at the smartphone level is expected within 2 years.

Acknowledgements. This work was supported, in part, by Grants of RFBR, Russia № 16-29-12998, 16-07-01140, 16-07-01047.

References

1. http://regulation.gov.ru/projects#npa=46657
2. Natenzon, M., Sokolov, I., Starodubov, V. et al.: Russian telemedicine consortium and the international telemedicine society BRICS. In: Forum International Society for Telemedicine & eHealth, Proceedings, Luxemburg, pp. 15–20 (2017)
3. Shklovsky-Kordi, N., Zingerman, B., Shifrin, M., Borodin, R., Shestakova, T., Vorobiev, A.: Engaging patients, empowering doctors in digitalization of healthcare. In: Siuly, S., et al. (eds.) HIS 2017. LNCS, vol. 10594, pp. 40–44. Springer, Cham (2017). https://doi.org/10.1007/978-3-319-69182-4_5
4. Shklovskiy-Kordi, N.E., Zingerman, B.: The protection of personal information and the patient's interests and safety - Russian experience. In: Proceedings ESH, Jerusalem, p. 84 (2010)
5. Gusev, A.V.: Criteria for choosing a medical information system (Rus.). Health Manag. **5**, 38–45 (2010)
6. Shklovskiy-Kordi, N., et al.: Intellectual algorithms for inspiring participation of the patient in a remote monitoring. In: STC 2017 Conference the Practice of Patient Centered Care, 23–24 October 2017, Tel Aviv, Israel (2017)

Author Index

Printed in the United States
By Bookmasters